Transdiagnostic Multiplex CBT for Muslim Cultural Groups

Transdiagnostic Multiplex CBT for Muslim Cultural Groups

Treating Emotional Disorders

Devon E. Hinton
Harvard Medical School

Baland Jalal
University of Cambridge

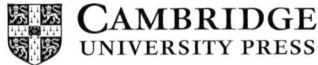

CAMBRIDGE
UNIVERSITY PRESS

University Printing House, Cambridge CB2 8BS, United Kingdom

One Liberty Plaza, 20th Floor, New York, NY 10006, USA

477 Williamstown Road, Port Melbourne, VIC 3207, Australia

314–321, 3rd Floor, Plot 3, Splendor Forum, Jasola District Centre,
New Delhi – 110025, India

79 Anson Road, #06–04/06, Singapore 079906

Cambridge University Press is part of the University of Cambridge.

It furthers the University's mission by disseminating knowledge in the pursuit of
education, learning, and research at the highest international levels of excellence.

www.cambridge.org
Information on this title: www.cambridge.org/9781108712798
DOI: 10.1017/9781108671217

First published 2020

Printed in the United Kingdom by TJ International Ltd, Padstow Cornwall

A catalogue record for this publication is available from the British Library.

Library of Congress Cataloging-in-Publication Data
Names: Hinton, Devon E., author. | Jalal, Baland, author.
Title: Transdiagnostic multiplex CBT for Muslim cultural groups : treating emotional disorders / Devon
E. Hinton, Baland Jalal.
Description: Cambridge ; New York, NY : Cambridge University Press, 2020. | Includes bibliographic
references and index.
Identifiers: LCCN 2020009232 (print) | LCCN 2020009233 (ebook) | ISBN 9781108712798 (paperback) |
ISBN 9781108671217 (ebook)
Subjects: LCSH: Muslims – Mental health – Western countries. | Muslims – Mental health services –
Western countries. | Psychotherapy – Religious aspects – Islam. | Cognitive therapy. | Stress (Psychology) –
Treatment. | Cross-cultural counseling.
Classification: LCC RC451.4.M87 H56 2020 (print) | LCC RC451.4.M87 (ebook) | DDC 616.890088/297–dc23
LC record available at https://lccn.loc.gov/2020009232
LC ebook record available at https://lccn.loc.gov/2020009233

ISBN 978-1-108-71279-8 Paperback

Contents

Introduction to Transdiagnostic Multiplex CBT for Muslim Cultural Groups

In spite of the popularity of cognitive behavior therapy (CBT) and much evidence supporting its overall efficacy (e.g., Blanchard, 2003; Cohen, Mannarino, & Murray, 2011; see also, Foa et al., 2008), there are few culturally sensitive CBT treatments available for Muslim cultural groups. There are currently around 1.6 billion Muslims in the world (a number expected to rise to 2.2 billion by the year 2030), with about 3.5 million Muslims living in the United States and 2.5 million in the United Kingdom (Pew Research Center, 2013). Additionally, given social and political unrest in the Middle East, Western countries (e.g., Europe, North America, and Australia) are likely to see an influx of Muslim refugees and immigrants in future years, many of whom suffer from mental disorders, including anxiety (e.g., post-traumatic stress disorder [PTSD]) and depressive disorders. There are also an increasing number of Muslims in the West currently finding themselves in need of therapeutic and social work services due to the negative impact of Islamophobic victimization, which likewise speaks to the pressing need for culturally sensitive treatments for this population.

Multiplex therapy as adapted for Muslim groups seeks to fill this gap by providing an accessible CBT treatment manual tailored primarily (but not exclusively) for Muslims living in the Western world (i.e., North America, Europe, as well as Australia), including immigrants and refugees, and other subgroups such as African Americans and second, third, and fourth generation American and European Muslims. The treatment manual is unique in that it takes into account the religious, spiritual, social, and cultural dimensions of individuals with a Muslim religious and/or cultural background. That is, the therapy frames treatment elements – that include mindfulness, loving-kindness meditation, attentional shifting, emotion regulation, yoga-like stretching, psychoeducation, anger management, and addressing catastrophic cognitions, pathological worry, and sleep-related problems (including sleep paralysis and nightmares) – in the context of well-known Islamic terms and concepts. Such cultural framing promotes treatment adherence and creates positive expectancy about treatment (Hinton & Jalal, in press), a major predictor of positive outcome in psychological research (e.g., Price, Finniss, & Benedetti, 2008). Indeed, culturally sensitive treatments have increased beneficial effects compared to non-adapted ones through the framing of treatment in terms of the patient's own understanding of disorder (Benish, Quintana, & Wampold, 2011).

Multiplex CBT has been shown to be effective for multiple cultural groups including Southeast Asian groups and South African tribes (Cambodian, Vietnamese, Sepedi) (Hinton, Pham et al., 2004; Hinton, Chhean et al., 2005; Hinton, Hofmann, Pollack et al., 2009; Hinton, Hofmann, Rivera et al., 2011; Jalal et al., in review) as well as multiple Muslim populations (Afghan, Egyptian, Syrian, and Turkish) (Acarturk, Abuhamdeh et al., 2019 Acarturk, Alyanak et al., in press; Jalal, Samir, & Hinton, 2017; Shaw et al., in press). Those

1

studies have demonstrated the efficacy of culturally adapted (CA) Multiplex CBT as compared to waitlist and applied muscle relaxation with large effect sizes similar to those resulting from traditional CBT. These studies have shown the efficacy of CA Multiplex CBT in both individual and group formats.[1]

Multiplex CBT takes into account issues like prominent somatic symptoms, low education, multiple comorbidities, ongoing life difficulties (e.g., financial stresses), and stigma about mental health, all of which are common challenges in Muslim populations and minority groups living in the West (Amer & Jalal, 2011; Jalal, Samir, & Hinton, 2017). Overall, Multiplex Therapy aims to be consistent with core Islamic beliefs, which may encourage this large population to seek treatment for their mental health problems. This is important, as there is often a distrust of mental health treatment among Muslims; psychotherapy and counselling, especially among first-generation immigrants, are seen as a secular science incongruent with basic Islamic values (Amir & Jalal, 2011). As such, this treatment manual is an important tool for therapists working in culturally diverse mental health settings.

Multiplex CBT as adapted for Muslim populations is also clinically relevant for non-Muslims. Indeed, its cultural framing could be considered as comparative examples that are used to better illustrate general therapeutic principles, as done with meditation and other Buddhist practices and principles, which are taught regardless of the religion of the individual in question. That is, showing how the treatment was adapted for Muslim populations illustrates general issues of adaptations as well as universal therapeutic principles, and the adaptation for a group of those universal principles.

Overview of Multiplex CBT

There are many obstacles when adapting standard CBT interventions (Foa & Rothbaum, 1998; Resick & Schnicke, 1996) to minority or cultural/religious groups. Such groups, including refugees and immigrants, may have low education, experience stigma about mental health and, crucially, have often undergone extensive traumas. As a result, standard treatment CBT techniques such as prolonged exposure for trauma may not be ideal for such groups, particularly those currently living in situations of stress and adversity (Hinton & Good, 2016; Hinton, Rivera et al., 2012), like those living in refugee centers and impoverished urban areas. Moreover, standard CBT does not make somatic symptoms a key therapeutic target and does not take into consideration that catastrophic cognitions about symptoms such as somatic symptoms, and comorbid conditions like worry, may vary across ethnic and cultural/religious groups (Hinton & Good 2016; Hinton, Rivera et al. 2012).

Multiplex CBT addresses many such challenges arising from working among refugee and minority populations (Hinton & Good, 2016; Hinton, Rivera et al., 2012). The key elements and overall session structure of Multiplex Therapy are shown in Table 1. For example, Multiplex CBT focuses on somatic symptoms and sensorial experiencing, as well as attentional processes, and stresses the importance of identifying and addressing key catastrophic cognitions that emerge from ethnopsychology and ethnospirituality such as catastrophic cognitions about "worry" and worry-induced symptoms; another

---

[1] All the treatment trials we have done have been with groups with minimal English ability and low education. The treatment techniques have been well accepted. As will be clear from the description of the treatment, its techniques have been designed to be easily understood by such groups.

Table 1 Sessions in Multiplex Therapy and key components of each session

Session Number	Session Title	Emotional Exposure Followed by Practice of the Indicated Protocol	Applied Stretching Lesson at Session's End	Mindfulness Lesson at Session's End
1	Education about Anxious-Depressive Distress and the Treatment and Introduction of Emotion Regulation Techniques	Anxious-Depressive Distress	X	X
2	Applied Stretching and the Toe-to-Head Muscle Relaxation with Visualization	Anxious-Depressive Distress	X	X
3	Review of Toe-to-Head Muscle Relaxation with Visualization and the Introduction of the Dysphoria (Anxiety/Depression) Protocol, Education about Anxious-Depressive Distress and Teaching the Bad Memory Protocol (Emotion Regulation Toolbox)	Anxious-Depressive Distress	X	X
4	Education about Anxious-Depressive Distress, Modifying Catastrophic Cognitions, and Teaching Emotional Distancing	Anxious-Depressive Distress	X	X
5	Interoceptive Exposure I: Head Rotation	Anxious-Depressive Distress	X	X

Table 1 (cont.)

Session Number	Session Title	Emotional Exposure Followed by Practice of the Indicated Protocol	Applied Stretching Lesson at Session's End	Mindfulness Lesson at Session's End
6	Interoceptive Exposure II: Hyperventilation	Anxious-Depressive Distress	X	X
7	Worry and Distress	Anxious-Depressive Distress	X	X
8	Anger and Anger Protocol, and Education about Breathing and Its Use for Relaxation	Anxious-Depressive Distress and Anger	X	X
9	Somatic Complaints and Sleep Disturbance	Anxious-Depressive Distress and Anger	X	X
10	Cultural Syndromes and Ethnophysiology Related to Distress	Anxious-Depressive Distress and Anger	X	X

focus is arousal and symptoms of arousal such as anger, which is a major treatment issue in cultural groups in stressful contexts (Hinton, Rasmussen et al., 2009).

Multiplex CBT is presented in an accessible way so that it can be administered both by highly trained clinicians (psychiatrists and clinical psychologists) and also by lesser-educated therapists. This is to ensure broader public health impact. The therapy is designed in a way that makes it accessible to patients with minimal or no schooling/education, which may be the case in refugee and immigrant populations and other lower-socio-economic status (SES) groups. To have wider public health impact (as dropout rates are typically high in minority groups such as among immigrants and refugees and other lower-SES communities), the treatment is relatively short, consisting of ten sessions (approximately one hour/session) that can be delivered once, twice, or three times a week, and can be administered to both individuals and groups of patients.

Multiplex CBT relies on a unique approach to exposure, with an emphasis on the emotion regulation of dysphoric states induced by asking about recent distressful memory recall and events. The patient is asked to describe such recall or other distressful events and then instructed to engage in emotion regulation techniques (i.e., what we call the Bad Memory Protocol [Emotion Regulation Toolbox], see Table 1) following the elicitation of distressing memories, including mindfulness, loving kindness, and applied muscle stretching with a visualization. It also includes interoceptive exposure to somatic sensations, many of which are thought to encode distressing events; the somatic distress cue is paired to a positive association (e.g., dizziness paired to positive memories of experiencing dizziness). Multiplex CBT uses yoga-like stretching and meditation techniques to promote emotional and psychological flexibility. It emphasizes the treatment of somatic sensations, targets comorbid anxiety conditions and anxiety-type psychopathological processes such as worry and panic attacks, and aims to reduce anger.

Finally, Multiplex Therapy is transdiagnostic in its approach, targeting anxiety and mood disorders, making it broad in its scope and applicable to a large segment of mental health patients. Such a transdiagnostic treatment also offers benefits such as ease of implementation (due to a decreased need for multiple manuals/treatments) and the possibility of providing group treatments to patients diagnosed with heterogeneous emotional disorders. The transdiagnostic therapeutic approach is increasingly being adopted as the preferred method of treatment, and as such is highly relevant to this cultural group.

We refer to the treatment as multiplex CBT because it targets multiple processes in our model of how anxious-depressive distress is generated, which is shown in Figure 1. As can be seen, the model emphasizes the role of somatic and mental symptoms, cultural understanding of symptoms, and emotion regulation processes. Our treatment targets processes in this model, as shall be discussed in more detail.

Cultural Framing for a Muslim Population

Culturally adapted Multiplex CBT takes into account the fact that Muslims living in the West have immigrated or may be the descendants of immigrants from a multiplicity of countries (e.g., Iraq, Syria, Turkey, Lebanon, Afghanistan, India, Pakistan, Bangladesh, and Somalia) and thus may represent, in some cases, diverse cultures. In America, there is, for instance, a strong presence of culturally distinct Muslim subgroups such as African American (approx. 20 percent of the US Muslim population) and, to a lesser extent, Caribbean Muslims. Similarly, there is a large group of Western Muslims who have converted into the faith. Although these groups may have unique cultural traditions, they all have in common basic Islamic beliefs as derived from the Quranic scripture and prophetic tradition (i.e., the "hadith literature"). This Islamic foundation should appeal across ethnicity, racial group, gender, SES, and age.

This approach of emphasizing basic Islamic teachings should appeal to persons from the various denominations of Islam. This includes major branches like Sunni (roughly 90 percent of all Muslims) and Shia (roughly 10 percent of all Muslims [often originating from Iran, Iraq, and Bahrain]). Whereas groups such as Sufi and Salafi (the latter prevalent in a Saudi Arabian context) are characterized by unique traditions in their own right, their teachings and practices broadly fall under the umbrella of Sunni Islam. It is worth pointing out that the hadith tradition, unlike Quranic scripture, may vary for Sunni and Shia Muslims. While Multiplex CBT refers to hadith literature derived from Sunni tradition (as noted, the largest Islamic denomination), the vast majority of Islamic references used in Multiplex CBT are quite basic and generally accepted and thus should appeal to all Muslims regardless of denomination.

Multiplex Therapy as adapted for Muslims aims to target heterogeneous Muslim populations by appealing to their underlying Islamic cultural heritage and belief systems. As an integral part of their culture, these group members would likely be familiar with basic Islamic concepts such as *salah* (ritualistic prayer that includes

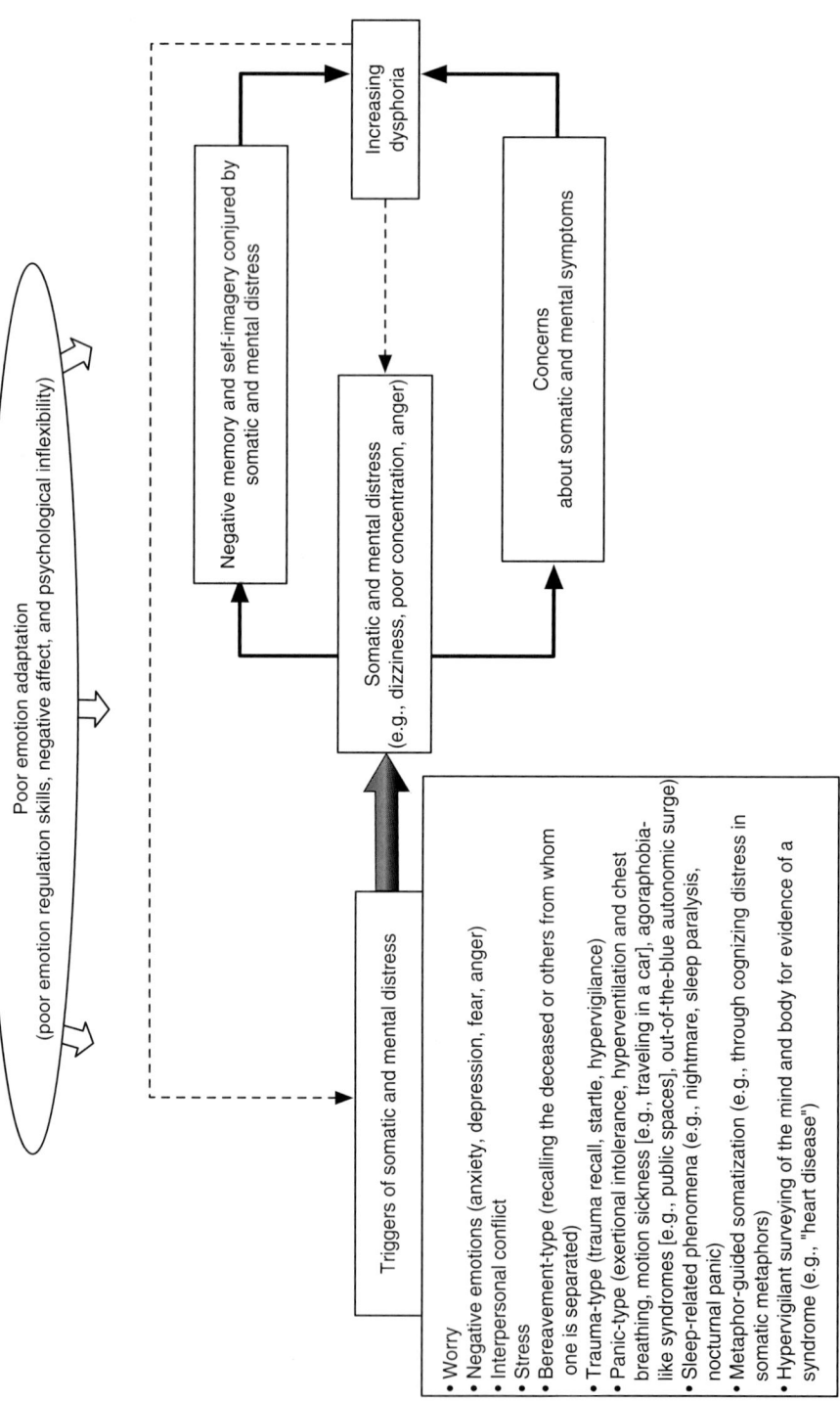

Figure 1. The Multiplex Model of the Generation of Anxious-Depressive Distress

bodily motions), *dua* (supplication, that is, asking God for various worldly favors or spiritual elevation and forgiveness), *fitra*[2] (one's natural or primordial state), *sadaqah* (charity), *tazkiyah*[3] (inner purification), *wudhu* and *ghusl* (ritualistic washing), *dhikr* (religious chanting as narrated in authentic hadith literature), *husnu dhun bilah* (having positive thoughts about Allah), *shukr* (gratefulness), *sunnah*[4] (prophetic customs and etiquettes), *haya* (chastity), *istighfar* (asking for forgiveness), *qadr* (predestination), and *asma-ul-husna* (Allah's 99 names as mentioned in the Quran). Members of such populations should readily identify with and accept well-known Quranic verses such as "Allah doesn't burden a soul beyond its capacity" (Quran 2:286) and "in the remembrance of God the hearts find rest" (Quran 13:28); prophetic sayings (e.g., "smiling in the face of your brother is charity"[5]) and narrations that emphasize the importance of cheerfulness and optimism; and stories of the prophets, for example, those of Yusuf (Joseph), Yacub (Jacob), and Ayub (Job), who remained optimistic, grateful and patient in spite of facing much adversity. Such cultural and religious terms, concepts, and parables are incorporated into the therapy thereby making it potentially more culturally consonant, acceptable, and relatable. In short, culturally adapted Multiplex CBT for Muslim populations emphasizes basic Islamic terms and concepts, thus making it accessible and relevant to Muslims of various ethnic and cultural backgrounds.

Nonetheless, regardless of the general appeal of Multiplex CBT's cultural adaptation, clinicians working with Muslim patients should always be flexible vis-à-vis religious adaptation. These must be personalized to the individual client's needs and background. Ideally, such a personalized approach would entail an initial assessment (e.g., in the form of an open dialog during the intake) about the patient's level of religiosity and cultural background (e.g., whether the patient is an African-American convert from Detroit versus a recent refugee from war-torn Syria) (see also, e.g., Amer & Jalal, 2011). By so doing, the therapist is able to better determine how much to emphasize and how to frame religious/cultural adaptation. For patients who are not religious, the religious rephrasing may be used as an example to make the concepts more understandable.

Key Treatment Dimensions of Multiplex CBT and the Adaptation for Muslim Populations

Here we discuss key treatment dimensions of Multiplex CBT and their adaptation for Muslim populations.

---

[2] *Fitra* refers to man's innate nature with which all humans are born, believed to be intrinsically wholesome and good.

[3] *Tazkiyah* refers to the engaging in inner purification of the soul, considered a type of worship. The soul might be purified by various means including contemplating the majesty and beauty of God, abstaining from all sin, and asking God for guidance and mercy.

[4] The *sunnah* refers to the prophet Muhammad's sayings, doings, and customs, that is, his overall practice (e.g., how he used to worship). The *sunnah* thus constitutes the prophetic path to be followed by Muslims guiding people to the worship of God. Indeed, the prophet Muhammad is regarded as the role model for all Muslims to emulate.

[5] Narration found in the at-Tirmidhi collection.

Normalizing Treatment and Promoting Adherence and Positive Expectancy

One way to normalize the treatment and create positive associations and expectancy is to provide certain descriptions of the entire treatment and its specific elements, grounding these elements in terms of culturally salient practices and metaphors. For example, in Multiplex CBT, treatment is compared to the making of a special cultural dish that involves multiple culinary steps in order to promote positive expectancy and to teach patience about the timeframe of improvement. As Muslims living in the West often have migrated from a multiplicity of countries with unique cultures and cuisines, one can refer to a special dish from the patient's culture, for example, by directly asking the patient about such cultural foods. This metaphor naturalizes treatment and teaches the patient that the treatment process takes multiple steps and requires patience, as does cooking. Thus, such metaphors that emphasize the need to complete all parts of the treatment, like those in which all elements of the treatment are analogized to the myriad steps needed to prepare a dish, may help increase credibility, positive expectancy, and tolerability, and address structural barriers.

As another way to increase overall adherence to the treatment, the therapist may similarly highlight the numerous verses from the Quran and sayings of prophet Muhammad stressing the importance of being patient in order to achieve one's goals (examples will be provided in the sessions that follow). In addition, as noted previously, Multiplex CBT frames CBT techniques in terms of Islamic healing traditions, thereby normalizing the process of treatment and increasing acceptance and positive expectancy. Examples include doing *dhikr* (i.e., engaging in the remembrance of Allah) to change attentional focus to a positive attentional object by engaging in the consecutive articulating of different names of God, which embodies attentional shift and a kind of descriptive flexibility, a viewing of an "object" from different perspectives.

Cultural Education about Anxious-Depressive Distress: The Inner Child

Educating patients about the anxiety-depressive state and psychopathological distress is another key part of Multiplex CBT. To this end, we use the metaphor of the "inner child" (an analogy for the brain's limbic system). This is a way of analogizing a distress state and its resolution to a common daily-life event; that is, using a disturbance-and-resolution analogy, a grounding image of emotion regulation. It helps to attain distance from the negative state and mobilize self-soothing capacities. It is also an opportunity to teach emotion regulation techniques. The inner child metaphor is introduced in the following way, using the example of negative memory or an upsetting event. We explain that an inner child keeps thinking about the distressing event(s), is continually frightened by it, and that this inner child, when reminded of the past, causes one to have strong emotions, such as feeling angry or sad, or somatic symptoms such as a fast-beating heart and so on. We then suggest that this inner child needs to be soothed.

For a Muslim population, the therapist can suggest soothing the child by using *dhikr* (which literally means "remembrance" in the Arabic language and in this context refers to the remembrance of Allah's names and attributes). *Dhikr* entails chanting religious phrases, for example, evoking and contemplating the meaning of different names for God. According to the Islamic faith, God has many names (an infinite number). Some of these were revealed to the prophet Muhammad, such as *ar-Rahman* (the Most Gracious), *ar-Raheem* (the Most

Table 2 Examples of names of Allah to reduce distress

	Name of Allah	Meaning
1.	*Ar-Rahman*	The Most Gracious
2.	*Ar-Raheem*	The Most Merciful
3.	*As-Salam*	The Provider of Peace
4.	*Al-Ghaffaar*	The Ever-Forgiving
5.	*Al-Wahhaab*	The Bestower
6.	*Ar-Razzaaq*	The Sustainer
7.	*Al-Mu'izz*	The Giver of Honor
8.	*Al-Latif*	The Most Kind
9.	*Al-Khabir*	The All-Aware
10.	*Al-Hafiz*	The Protector
11.	*Al-Muqit*	The Nourisher
12.	*Al-Karim*	The Most Generous
13.	*Al-Mujib*	The Responsive
14.	*Al-Wadud*	The Most Loving
15.	*Al-Wali*	The Protecting Friend

Note: While the names of Allah may be evoked at any given time, they can also be evoked depending on one's circumstance. A person in need of protection may evoke the name *al-Wali* (the Protecting Friend), the person who craves inner peace the name *as-Salam* (the Provider of Peace), and the person worrying about financial difficulties the name *ar-Razaaq* (the Bestower).

Merciful), *al-Wadood* (the Ever-Most Loving), *al-Mumin* (the Granter of Security), *al-Muhaymin* (the Protector), *al-Salam* (the Ultimate Provider of Peace), *al-Muqit* (the Nourisher), and *al-Gafur* (the Forgiving). In this regard, one may mention to the patient that the Quran (Islam's holy book) encourages Muslims to call upon God using these different names (see verse 17:110–111), and that he or she may evoke these names of God to soothe the inner child (see Table 2 for selected names for God). Also, one can mention how this child is safe and protected in the presence of God. A special *dhikr* that a patient may say to soothe the inner child is repeating each of three distinct praises of God – *subhanAllah* (glory be to God; thirty-three times), *alhamdulilah* (praise be to God; thirty-three times), *Allahuakbar* (God is the greatest; thirty-four times) – all the while using his or her fingers to count (called *tasbeeh*). Also, the clinician can mention to the patient the following verse in the Quran, in which God says, "in the remembrance of God the hearts find rest" (Quran: 13:28), a reassurance that the *dhikr* may bring inner peace and comfort to the "inner child."

It is important to note that this inner child analogy should be used cautiously when working with male Muslim patients. In our pilot work in Egypt using this metaphor, we found that a subset of Muslim Arab males found it somewhat problematic. This is probably because the idea of rocking an inner child may go against conventional Arab ideals stressing male masculinity. Many Muslims living in Western countries originate from Middle Eastern or Asian societies with similar ideals of masculinity (the same may be the case for African-American Muslims and second and third generation European Muslims including converts, originating from inner city and urban areas). As an alternative to the inner child metaphor, the clinician could refer simply to the "inner part of oneself," which we have found to be more appropriate in an Arab/Muslim Egyptian context.

Teaching Mindfulness and Attentional Control

Mindfulness meditation techniques are an integral part of many types of CBT (i.e., the so-called third wave of behavior therapies: Hayes, Strosahl, & Wilson, 1999; Linehan, 1993; Segal, Williams, & Teasdale, 2002). Such techniques include being mindful of sensorial experiencing and acceptance of negative internal sensations and thoughts as opposed to trying to change them through an observational mindset (Brown, Gaudiano, & Miller, 2011; Herbert, Forman, & England, 2009). More generally, mindfulness involves being aware of the current attentional focus and learning to distance from that attentional focus in order to select a certain attentional focus (e.g., taking the mind away from worry to attend to the breath). We consider mindfulness and attentional control to be closely related. We will consider mindfulness in a broad sense as the taking of a certain attentional object with a certain emotional and/or cognitive frame so that it includes, for example, attending to the breath, attending to ambient nature, and loving kindness. (The mindful taking on of a certain attentional object with a certain frame that may be emotional, cognitive, and bodily; a certain emotion-cognitive-body set.)

Multiplex CBT teaches the importance of attentional focus. For instance, how the attentional object determines mood, and the fleeting nature of mood. It teaches techniques to help patients attend to the sensorial experience of the current environmental surrounding and to the body itself, and to notice the mood change that happens when shifting the mind from rumination to attending to the surrounding visual scape – leaves moving in the wind, for instance. It uses religious-based strategies derived from Islamic tradition to promote attentional-shifting, and to teach the patient to move the mind away from worries to a positive attentional object. For example, as ways to shift attention and to teach how the attentional object shapes mood, we recommend *dhikr,* such as the practice of remembering and evoking the names of God (usually while moving just the tongue without producing any vocal tract sound) and contemplating their deeper meanings. See Table 2 and the following sessions for various ways to do *dhikr* that include *tasbeeh*; reciting the Quran (Islam's holy book); engaging in *dua* (supplication, e.g., while evoking God's names and attributes); and engaging in *salah* (a ritualistic form of prayer where the individual prostrates, bows, and stands).

We integrate into treatment the practice of *salah,* which entails attentional focus and performing bodily stretching. As such, it is a way to embody flexibility (analogous to yoga). It is simultaneously a method to shift emotional focus to a positive object, to promote a low-impact physical activity (a type of "behavioral activation"), and to break vicious cycles of inactivity and inertia (e.g., sedentary habits that are exacerbated by psychopathology). As *salah* is to be performed throughout the day (five times per day) within specified time periods (morning, noon, afternoon, evening, and night), it is ideal for breaking sedentary habits. During *salah,* while uttering praises of God, the person bows down in a 90-degree angle and then stretches out on the ground with his or her face pointing downwards. Worshippers are encouraged to remain in these positions for as long as possible. They are indeed regarded as among the highest acts of worship (referred to in Arabic as *sajdah* and *rukuh*). The idea is to do *salah* with utmost attentional focus and emotional centeredness – that is, to enter into a meditative state, called *kushoo* in Arabic, with complete focus on God (e.g., on His infinite mercy and glory). This is a form of concentration meditation. Prophet Muhammad, the role model for Muslims, would himself regularly spend hours at night in this meditative state; this included long periods of stretching out with his face pressed on the ground or his body in a bowing position, while chanting God's praises, or standing straight while reciting the Quran (see "Sahih Al-Bukhari," book 19, hadith 2, the foremost authoritative work after the Quran). In this example, there is an element of embodied flexibility, somatic mode of attention (i.e., on bodily stretches), and focused attention on God, combined with the overall satisfaction of pleasing the deity resulting in further positive affect. Multiplex CBT includes bodily stretching paired to flexibility metaphors (Hinton, Rivera et al., 2012). It is thus ideal to mention *salah* in the context of stretching exercises.

All religious acts (e.g., those mentioned) performed by Muslims require what is called *kushoo*, namely, absolute attentional focus and "God awareness." Such focused attention is emphasized in Multiplex CBT to amplify mindfulness. During treatment, it is clarified to patients that attending to positive objects, such as to God during prayer, dictates mood and emotion. As such, fully focusing on God's infinite mercy and glory during *salah*, *dua*, and *dhikr*, is therapeutically beneficial.

Multiplex CBT teaches a specific meditation technique called "loving kindness" aiming to improve positive affect and attentional focus (see Hinton, Ojserkis et al., 2013; Hinton, Pich, Hofmann, & Otto, 2013). For a Muslim population, patients are told to direct love to God first (a type of ultimate love) and thereafter to his prophets; next to other human beings, starting with the *ummah* (the global Muslim community) and then to all mankind; and lastly to himself or herself. This particular hierarchy of directing loving kindness is more in line with core Islamic values, with God deserving a form of ultimate love. Prophets are next in line as they belong to the spiritual realm and deserve a type of spiritual and transcendent love and admiration. Next, selfless love is directed to others, including family members, which is crucial according to Islam; a type of a non-ego-based love. Such love should ideally first be directed towards parents, starting with the mother and then the father (and then remaining family members). This is in line with the Quranic ethos of parental love, which is highly prized. That is, in several verses the Quran stresses the importance of supplicating for one's parents and showing them mercy, especially the mother; for instance, "and lower to them [i.e., your parents] the wing of humility out of mercy and say, 'My Lord, have mercy upon them as they brought me up [when I was] small,'" (17:24), and "We [i.e., God] have enjoined upon man [to take good care] of his parents. His mother carried him, [increasing her] in weakness upon weakness, and his weaning is in two years. Be grateful to Me [i.e., God] and to your parents" (31:14). We tell patients to direct love towards the *ummah* (the global Muslim community) and then all mankind. Again, this order of showing love and kindness is consistent with the Prophet's teachings that Muslims globally belong to a special brotherhood/sisterhood. This type of emphasis on collectivistic/social empathic bonding is echoed in his statements such as, "none of you has faith until he loves for his brother or neighbor what he loves for himself,"[6] and advice to his followers to make *dua* (e.g., supplicate) for one another, as so doing would make the

---

[6] See Sahih al-Bukhari.

angels in the sky make *dua* for the supplicating person in return.[7] Such collectivistic empathy is not restricted to the *ummah* (Muslim community) but indeed is for all mankind, as the Prophet noted, "Allah will not be merciful to those who are not merciful to mankind."[8] Indeed, given prophet Muhammad's emphasis on supplicating for others, such loving-kindness meditation may conclude by recommending that the patient supplicate for himself and others if he so wishes (e.g., asking for forgiveness, i.e., repenting, in Arabic referred to as making *tauba*).

In Islamic tradition, water and cooling imagery is highly valued, which is incorporated into the loving-kindness visualization. The Quran narrates the story of the prophet Job (*Ayub*, in Arabic) who fell ill and was eventually instructed by God to strike the ground with his foot. This, in turn, caused cool, healing waters to gush forth from the earth for him to drink and bathe in. Job thus became cured of his sickness (Quran 38:41–43). Likewise, the prophet Abraham was thrown into a fire, but miraculously survived as sudden coldness from God covered his body, "oh fire be you coolness and safety for Abraham" (Quran 21:69). During piloting of Multiplex CBT, we found such cooling imagery to work well with Muslim populations, and these specific prophetic examples may be mentioned when referring to this imagery.

Multiplex CBT utilizes facial-expression mindfulness. This may entail exhibiting a slight smile in social situations. We have found this to improve mood overall and strengthen the person's interpersonal and social bonds. To encourage frequent smiling habits, we stress that smiling was recommended by the prophet Muhammad, who is the role model for all Muslims to emulate as per the Quran, "surely there was a good example for you in the Messenger of Allah (i.e., prophet Muhammad [33:21]). Prophet Muhammad was seen smiling often,[9] and notably said that "smiling in the face of your brother is charity."[10]

Another cultural way to teach mindfulness and present-moment sensorial awareness is via the Islamic concept of "mindful eating." The prophet Muhammad said that "when one of you eats some food, let him say *Bismillah* (i.e., in the name of God),"[11] and also taught his followers to praise Allah upon finishing eating; for instance, "Allah is pleased with His servant [or slave] when he eats something and praises Him for it, or drinks something and praises Him for it."[12] This is a way to teach attentional focus, mindfulness, and gratitude as applied to a seemingly trivial (reoccurring) everyday life-event, namely eating. Furthermore, the Prophet emphasized the importance of not overeating; for example, he said, "a man does not fill any vessel worse than his stomach."[13] This is another approach to addressing mindless habitual eating, by being acutely aware of one's food intake. To further encourage patients to adopt mindful eating habits, the therapist may remind the patient of the overall benefits of not overeating (e.g., increased energy and health benefits like weight loss and reduced bodily inflammation implicated in psychopathology [Su, 2012].) Similarly, the concept of fasting (associated with numerous health benefits like neuronal autophagy [e.g., Alirezaei et al., 2010]) may be recommended to patients as a way to promote mindful eating and gratitude upon breaking the fast. Many Muslims, with the exception of the frail, sick, and elderly, fast (i.e., abstain from food and water consumption) from sunrise to sunset for an entire month each year (i.e., the month of *ramadhan*, which is one of the five pillars of Islam). However, voluntary fasting may

---

[7] See Sahih Muslim.   [8] See Sahih al-Bukhari.
[9] Narrations on the Prophet smiling often are available in al-Bukhari and Muslim collection.
[10] Narration found in the at-Tirmidhi collection.
[11] Narration found in the at-Tirmidhi collection.   [12] Found in the Muslim collection.
[13] Narration found in the at-Tirmidhi collection.

be done year-round, and the Prophet himself often used to fast Mondays and Thursdays.[14] Such acts of fasting may foster a sense of appreciation and gratitude for food and enhance mindful eating once the fast is broken; having been deprived of food for many hours, the person may become more perceptive of the rich flavors and smells of food, its texture, and so on. We attempt to augment such sensorial experiencing by asking the patient to eat such fast-breaking meals while concentrating on the flavors, smells, appearance, touch, and even sound of chewing and swallowing. This is a way to counteract mindless habitual eating and transform the act of eating into an enhanced present-moment sensorial experience.

Multiplex CBT aims to further promote present-moment sensorial awareness of the environment. To teach this to Muslim patients, we suggest that patients contemplate the beauty of God's creation, like watching the clouds, the greenery of trees, and the leaves moving gently with the wind (which is yet another way to teach flexibility, promoting emotion regulation). As a way to anchor such present-moment sensorial awareness in the Islamic cultural frame, the therapist can highlight Quranic verses on the topic of appreciating the beauty of nature (God's creation): "this is the creation of God. So show Me what those other than Him have created" (31:11), "[such is] the artistry of God [i.e., referring to the creation], who perfected all things" (27:88), and "[God] perfected everything which He created" (32:7).

Finally, one cultural healing practice encouraged by Multiplex CBT involves attentional focus (concentration meditation) and positive bodily self-awareness, a practice called *ruqyah*. It entails recitation of Quranic verses to promote bodily healing (Hinton & Jalal, 2014). For example, during *ruqyah*, the person may recite Quranic verses and then gently blow on various parts of his or her own body, or over a bucket of water used for drinking or bathing, or even over an olive oil container (it is not uncommon to massage such olive oil on the body prior to sleep [the olive is regarded as a blessed food in Islamic culture as too in the biblical tradition]). These cultural practices promote attentional focus and emotion centeredness and bodily relaxation, including release of muscle tension (see too Amer & Jalal, 2011). They function as body-focused emotion regulation techniques.

Addressing Sleep-Related Issues

Multiplex CBT targets sleep and sleep-related phenomena such as nightmares, sleep paralysis, and nocturnal panic. It does so through various means, including yoga-like stretching before sleeping to decrease tension and arousal (as well as promoting psychological flexibility) and shifting nightmare content upon awakening from sleep. Culturally specific techniques may be recommended in addition to standard CBT interventions for disturbed sleep. Islamic tradition has a number of such practices that Multiplex CBT encourages (see Table 3).

In many non-Western cultures, nightmares are regarded as the visitation of a deceased person or other dangerous being (Hinton, Hinton et al., 2009). In Islamic culture, nightmares are thought to be inspired by evil spirits (*shayateen*), whereas good dreams or visions (*mubashiraat* in Arabic) are inspired by God through His angels. Patients are reminded that Islam teaches that one should ignore nightmares, and avoid talking about them to others, as these in essence are meaningless (have no substance and only cause unnecessary fear and worry). The patient, after a terrifying nightmare, could ask God for refuge and inner peace, and even do *salah* as the prophet Muhammad advised his followers, to reduce any associated distress.

---

[14] Narration found in the at-Tirmidhi collection.

Table 3 Islamic-based sleep practices to employ before sleeping and upon awakening that are used in the CA-CBT sleep module (see too Jalal, Samir, & Hinton, 2017)

Before sleeping	Upon awakening from sleep
1. Perform *wudhu* (ritualistic washing)	1. Perform *salah-tul-subh* (the morning prayer)
2. Pray *witr* (night prayer)	2. Recite *dua* (supplications) recommended by the prophet Muhammad
3. Recite Quranic verses (112; 113; 114) and/or chapter 2 verse 255 (i.e., *Ayah Al-Kursi*) and/or chapter 67 (*Al-Mulk*)	
4. Chant *tasbeeh* (praises of God)	
5. Recite *dua* (supplications) recommended by the prophet Muhammad	

Note. Wudhu refers to the ritualistic washing of the body including the hands, face, and feet. *Witr* is a special *salah* that in the Islamic religion is specifically only performed before going to sleep at night. The Quranic verses 112, 113, and 114 are thought to bring about God's protection from devils that might harm the sleeper. *Tasbeeh* is a form of *dhikr* (religious chanting) in which the person chants praises to God; *tasbeeh* may include saying, *subhanAllah* (glory be to God; thirty-three times), *alhamdulilah* (praise be to God; thirty-three times), and *Allahuakbar* (God is the greatest; thirty-four times), using the fingers to count. In respect to *dua*, the prophet Muhammad recommended many *dua* (supplications) before sleeping; see Hisnul Muslim by Sa'id bin Ali Ibn Wahf Al-Qahtaani. For instance, one could say, "In your Name, Oh God, I die and live" (*bismika allahumma amootu wa ahya*). *Salah-tul-subh* is a ritualistic prayer (or *salah*) that in the Islamic religion is performed early in the morning upon awakening from sleep. The prophet Muhammad recommended many *dua* (supplications) upon awakening from sleep; for instance, one could say, "All praise is to God who gave us life after death [death here refers to sleep that is considered a minor form of death in Islam] and to Him is the resurrection" (*alhamdulillahil-ladhee ahyana ba'da maa amaatana wa ilayhin-nushoor*) (see Hisnul Muslim).

Addressing Worry

Uncontrollable worry is a central part of the distress pathology among refugees, ethnic populations, and treatment seekers in general (Hinton, Rivera et al., 2012). Common worry themes include financial stressors, health issues, housing issues, and residing in dangerous localities with sociopolitical instability. Multiplex CBT elicits worry topics that are of great concern. This process facilitates an empathic bond between patient and therapist (the patient feels understood) that improves the therapeutic alliance overall. Ideally, worry topics can be addressed. Also, Multiplex CBT reframes worry-type distress in adaptive imagery and metaphors that help to regulate distress, and it promotes present-moment mindfulness, the use of culturally relevant emotion regulation techniques, and the experiencing of certain emotions (e.g., gratitude) as adaptive mindsets to address worry. There is a shift from a maladaptive to an adaptive mindset (on gratitude as an adaptive emotional state, see Wood, Froh, & Geraghty, 2010).

Multiplex CBT as applied to Muslim populations refers to traditional Islamic practices when teaching ways to alleviate worry and improve emotional regulation and decrease other types of negative affect. This includes encouraging the patient to engage in any supplication (*dua*) recommended by prophet Muhammad to reduce worry and anxiety states. For example, the patient may recite the following supplication when in a distressed state, "Oh the Living, oh the Eternal, I seek help in Your grace" (*ya hayyu, ya qayyumu, bi-rahmatika astaghithu*)[15]. The patient may also consider doing *salah* (ritualistic prayer) or reciting *dhikr* (chanting different praises of Allah).

One cognitive reframing technique we use to foster optimism is reminding the patient of the idea of *qadr* (i.e., divine predestination, one of the six major pillars of Islamic beliefs, *arkan al iman*; not to be confused with the five pillars of Islam: *arkan al Islam*). It may be said to the patient that according to *qadr*, worrying will not change what God has predetermined, and will therefore not alter current circumstances. The patient is encouraged to instead engage in *dua* (supplication, as discussed previously) to counter negative affective states; as the prophet Muhammad famously said according to one narration, "nothing can change Divine Decree except *dua* [supplication]."[16] Thus, *dua* provides a psychologically positive tool to channel frustration and worry. Likewise, the patient is encouraged to have positive expectations for the future and think positively about God (*husnu dhun bilah*), being grateful for the present (*shukr*), irrespective of one's condition. According to Islamic tradition, optimism about God (i.e., which indirectly affirms God's infinitely merciful nature) and displaying gratefulness for the present (*shukr*), are ways to increase one's blessings (the hadith regarding *husnu dhun bilah* is found in the *Sahih Al-Bukhari* collection, and on *shukr* vis-à-vis increasing blessing, see Quran 14:7).

One can additionally refer to Quranic stories that evoke this theme. For example, prophet Jacob (in Arabic *Yaqub*), prophet Joseph (in Arabic *Yusuf*), and prophet Job (in Arabic *Ayub*) are depicted in the Quran as going through major trials and tribulations. But, because of their high level of gratefulness in spite of circumstances (*shukr*) and their positive expectations of God (*husnu dhun bilah*), they were eventually rewarded by God.

Another key Quranic principle to help cope with worry and distress is the concept of *tawakkul* – that is, putting one's trust fully in Allah (i.e., trusting in Allah's overarching plan). This is a fundamental Islamic theme, heavily evoked in the Quran (i.e., numerous verses); for example, "Allah loves those who put their trust in him" (3:159), and "put your trust in the All-Mighty, the Most Merciful (i.e., Allah)" (see Hamdan, 2008; see too Amer & Jalal, 2011). The *tawakkul* mindset entails a full reliance on God regardless of circumstance, a firm conviction that God is the one who is in control of all things in the universe, and trust that God's help and assistance will eventually be granted to those who have *tawakkul* (those who rely on God). This Quranic concept is meant to eradicate worry and anxiety, and teach resilience in the face of adversity, because the person submits his affairs to God, trusting that all will be well in the end (of note, submitting to the will of God aligns with the very definition of the word *Islam*, highlighting the central role of *tawakkul* in the Islamic faith).

Tawakkul is closely related to the notion of *ibtilah* (trial or tribulation). The Quran mentions, "We will surely test you with something of fear and hunger and a loss of wealth and lives and fruits, but give good tidings to the patient" (2:155). This is the idea that each person will be tested by God in various ways (i.e., will inevitably go through trial and tribulation); but that trusting in God, asking God for forgiveness (i.e., repenting, in Arabic making *tauba*) and having patience, is the way to pass such tests, leading to a state of inner peace. As noted, during therapy, one could mention the examples of the Islamic prophets (e.g., Abraham, Moses, Jesus, and Muhammad) who were tested by God but eventually were aided out of their troubles because of their *tawakkul* mindset. A potent way to engender such *tawakkul* in the face of life's adversities is to remind the patient that whenever a person goes through any hardship (e.g., poverty, loss of a loved one, sickness) sins are erased

---

[15] See Hisnul Muslim.   [16] See at-Tirmidhi collection.

accordingly. Indeed, such adversities are a means whereby the person will be forgiven by God and become spiritually elevated (i.e., akin to the prophets). In this vein, prophet Muhammad taught, "There is no calamity that befalls a Muslim but Allah expiates (sin) thereby, even a thorn that pricks him."[17] In another narration, the Prophet said (in the context of illness but with a general meaning), "No Muslim is afflicted with any harm but that Allah will remove his sins as the leaves of a tree fall down."[18] This principle (emotional reshifting strategy) is a way to pair negative life events (and the negative emotions they elicit such as distress and worry) with a positive occurrence (God's forgiveness and spiritual elevation).

Teaching Anger Management

Anger is also a major treatment focus of Multiplex CBT (Hinton, Rasmussen et al., 2009; Hinton, Rivera et al., 2012). There are a number of ways to frame anger management to make it culturally targeted for a Muslim population. For example, the clinician may tell the patient that Islam stresses that anger should be avoided. Prophet Muhammad emphasized that true strength is not physical strength (i.e., muscular) but successfully controlling one's anger; he advised his followers, "do not become angry."[19] Similarly, the Prophet advised his followers that, "when one of you becomes angry while standing, he should sit down. If the anger leaves him, well and good; otherwise he should lie down"[20] (see also, Amer & Jalal, 2011). This is a form of anger management technique that minimizes the likelihood that the person will engage in undesirable behavior during anger outbursts that will later be regretted. Other techniques include doing *wudhu* (ritualistic washing of the face and limbs) and physically leaving the location where one became angry (Haque, 2004; Amer & Jalal, 2011).

Culturally Indicated Transitional Rituals

Multiplex CBT encourages patients to make use of transitional rites at the end of therapy as a way to increase positive self-imagery and expectancy about treatment. We specifically recommend the purification ritual known as *wudhu*. This is ritualistic washing of the face, arms, and feet. The act of *wudhu* is mandatory preparation for *salah* (ritualistic prayer), and is recommended before any act of worship such as making *dua* (supplication) and before sleeping; and also, when feeling angry, to cool down (see previous section on anger management). Islam teaches that during *wudhu*, any body part that comes in contact with water is cleansed of sin. For instance, by rinsing the mouth, it is cleansed from any sins, such as profanities uttered during the course of the day. We also recommend the related act called *ghusl*, which is the ritualistic washing of the entire body. *Ghusl* is a greater and more extensive form of spiritual and physical purification. It is performed after sexual intercourse (i.e., prior to *salah*), after menstrual periods for women, and ideally before going to the mosque on Fridays or religious festivities, and also after religious conversion. Both *wudhu* and *ghusl* are forms of attentional training: Muslims are encouraged to be mindful of God during *wudhu* and *ghusl* and they are in a somatic mood of attention (viz., with bodily cleansing, such as water running down the limbs and cleansing off sins). *Wudhu* and *ghusl* are ways for the

---

[17] Found in al-Bukhari.   [18] Found in al-Bukhari.   [19] Found in al-Bukhari.
[20] In Sunan Abi Dawud.

person to transition into a symbolic state of spiritual purity, which is also free from physical impurity. As such, Multiplex CBT encourages patients to make use of *wudhu* and *ghusl* to promote a sense of closure and a feeling of transformation, including a change in self-image, and to foster positive expectancy about the completed treatment (Hinton et al., 2012).

References

Acarturk, C., Abuhamdeh, S., Jalal, B., et al. (2019). Culturally adapted transdiagnostic CBT for SSRI-resistant Turkish adolescents: A pilot study of group treatment. *American Journal of Orthopsychiatry, 89*, 222–227.

Acarturk, C., Alyanak, B., Cetinkaya, M., Gulen, B., Jalal, B., & Hinton, D. (in press). Adaptation of transdiagnostic CBT for Turkish adolescents: Examples from culturally adapted Multiplex CBT (CA Multiplex CBT). *Cognitive Behavioral Practice.*

Alirezaei, M., Kemball, C. C., Flynn, C. T., Wood, M. R., Whitton, J. L., & Kiosses, W. B. (2010). Short-term fasting induces profound neuronal autophagy. *Autophagy, 6*(6), 702–710.

Amer, M. & Jalal, B. (2011). Individual psychotherapy/counseling: Psychodynamic, cognitive behavioral and humanistic-experiential models. In Ahmed, S. & Amer, M. (Eds). *Counseling Muslims: Handbook of mental health issues and interventions.* New York: Routledge.

Benish, S. G., Quintana, S., & Wampold, B. E. (2011). Culturally adapted psychotherapy and the legitimacy of myth: A direct-comparison meta-analysis. *Journal of Counseling Psychology, 58*(3), 279–289.

Blanchard, E. B., Hickling, E. J., Devineni, T., Veazey, C. H., Galovski, T. E., Mundy, E., . . . & Buckley, T. C. (2003). A controlled evaluation of cognitive behaviorial therapy for posttraumatic stress in motor vehicle accident survivors. *Behaviour Research and Therapy, 41*(1), 79–96.

Brown, L. A., Gaudiano, B. A., & Miller, I. W. (2011). Investigating the similarities and differences between practitioners of second- and third-wave cognitive-behavioral therapies. *Behavior modification, 35*(2), 187–200.

Cohen, J. A., Mannarino, A. P., & Murray, L. K. (2011). Trauma-focused CBT for youth who experience ongoing traumas. *Child Abuse & Neglect, 35*(8), 637–646.

Foa, E. B., Keane, T. M., Friedman, M. J., & Cohen, J. A. (Eds.). (2008). *Effective treatments for PTSD: Practice guidelines from the International Society for Traumatic Stress Studies.* New York: Guilford Press.

Foa, E. B., & Rothbaum, B. O. (1998). Treating the trauma of rape: Cognitive-behavioral therapy for PTSD. New York: Guilford Press.

Hamdan, A. (2008). Cognitive restructuring: An Islamic perspective. *Journal of Muslim Mental Health, 3*, 99–116.

Haque, A. (2004). Religion and mental health: The case of American Muslims. *Journal of Religion and Health, 43*, 45–58.

Hayes, S. C., Strosahl, K. D., & Wilson, K. G. (1999). *Acceptance and commitment therapy: An experiential approach to behavior change.* New York: Guilford Press.

Herbert, J. D., Forman, E. M., England, E. L. (2009). Psychological acceptance. In O'Donohue, W., & Fisher, J. E. (Eds). *General principles and empirically supported techniques of cognitive behavior therapy.* Hoboken, NJ: John Wiley & Sons.

Hinton, D. E., Chhean, D., Pich, V., Safren, S. A., Hofmann, S. G., & Pollack, M. H. (2005). A randomized controlled trial of cognitive-behavior therapy for Cambodian refugees with treatment-resistant PTSD and panic attacks: A cross-over design. *Journal of Traumatic Stress, 18*(6), 617–629.

Hinton, D. E., & Good, B. J. (Eds.). (2016). *Culture and PTSD: Trauma in global and historical perspective.* Philadelphia: University of Pennsylvania Press.

Hinton, D. E., Hinton, A., Chhean, D., Pich, V., Loeum, J. R., & Pollack, M. H. (2009). Nightmares among Cambodian refugees: The breaching of concentric ontological security. *Culture, Medicine, and Psychiatry, 33*, 219–265.

Hinton, D. E., Hofmann, S. G., Pollack, M. H., & Otto, M. W. (2009). Mechanisms of efficacy of CBT for Cambodian refugees with PTSD: Improvement in emotion regulation and orthostatic blood pressure response. *CNS*

Neuroscience and Therapeutics, 15(3), 255–263.

Hinton, D. E., Hofmann, S. G., Rivera, E., Otto, M. W., & Pollack, M. H. (2011). Culturally adapted CBT for Latino women with treatment-resistant PTSD: A pilot study comparing CA-CBT to Applied Muscle Relaxation. *Behaviour Research and Therapy, 49*, 275–280.

Hinton, D. E., & Jalal, B. (2014). Parameters for creating culturally sensitive CBT: Implementing CBT in global settings. *Intervention, 203*(11), 871–875.

Hinton, D. E., & Jalal, B. (in press). Dimensions of culturally sensitive CBT: Application to Southeast Asian and other Asian populations. *American Journal of Orthopsychiatry.*

Hinton, D. E., Ojserkis, R. A., Jalal, B., Peou, S., & Hofmann, S. G. (2013). Loving-Kindness in the treatment of traumatized refugees and minority groups: A typology of mindfulness and the nodal network model of affect and affect regulation. *Journal of Clinical Psychology, 69*(8), 817–828.

Hinton, D. E., Pham, T., Tran, M., Safren, S. A., Otto, M. W., & Pollack, M. H. (2004). CBT for Vietnamese refugees with treatment-resistant PTSD and panic attacks: A pilot study. *Journal of Traumatic Stress, 17* (5), 429–433.

Hinton, D. E., Pich, V., Hofmann, S. G., & Otto, M. W. (2013). Mindfulness and acceptance techniques as applied to refugee and ethnic minority populations: Examples from culturally adapted CBT (CA-CBT). *Cognitive and Behavioral Practice, 20*, 33–46.

Hinton, D. E., Rasmussen, A., Nou, L., Pollack, M. H., & Good, M. J. (2009). Anger, PTSD, and the nuclear family: A study of Cambodian refugees. *Social Science and Medicine, 69*, 1387–1394.

Hinton, D. E., Rivera, E., Hofmann, S. G., Barlow, D. H., & Otto, M. W. (2012). Adapting CBT for traumatized refugees and ethnic minority patients: Examples from culturally adapted CBT (CA-CBT). *Transcultural Psychiatry, 49*, 340–365.

Jalal, B., Kruger, Q., & Hinton, D. (in review). Culturally Adapted CBT (CA-CBT) for traumatized indigenous South Africans (Sepedi): A randomized pilot trial comparing CA-CBT to applied muscle relaxation. *Intervention: Journal of Mental Health and Psychosocial Support in Conflict Affected Areas.*

Jalal, B., Samir, S. W., & Hinton, D. E. (2017). Adaptation of CBT for traumatized Egyptians: Examples from culturally adapted CBT (CA-CBT). *Cognitive and Behavioral Practice, 24*, 58–71.

Linehan, M. M. (1993). *Cognitive-behavioral treatment of borderline personality disorder.* New York: Guilford Press.

Pew Research Center (2013). World's Muslim population more widespread than you might think. https://www.pewresearch.org/fact-tank/2017/01/31/worlds-muslim-population-more-widespread-than-you-might-think/.

Price, D. D., Finniss, D. & Benedetti, F. (2008). A comprehensive review of the placebo effect: Recent advances and current thought. *Annual Review of Psychology. 59*, 565–590.

Resick, P., & Schnicke, M. (1996). *Cognitive processing therapy for rape victims.* London, UK: Sage.

Sahih al-Bukhari. Accessed September 19, 2014, from http://sunnah.com/bukhari/19.

Segal, Z. V., Williams, J. M. G., & Teasdale, J. D. (2002). *Mindfulness-based cognitive therapy for depression: A new approach to preventing relapse.* New York: Guilford Press.

Shaw, S. A., Ward, K. P., Pillai, V., & Hinton, D. E. (in press). A group mental health randomized controlled trial for female refugees in Malaysia. *American Journal of Orthopsychiatry.*

Su, K. P. (2012). Inflammation in psychopathology of depression: Clinical, biological, and therapeutic implications. *BioMedicine, 2*(2), 68–74.

Wood, A. M., Froh, J. J., & Geraghty, A. W. (2010). Gratitude and well-being: A review and theoretical integration. *Clinical Psychology Review, 30*(7), 890–905.

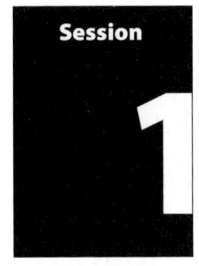

Education about Anxious-Depressive Distress and the Treatment and Introduction of Emotion Regulation Techniques

Overview of Core Lessons

The goal of this session is to briefly describe the goals of the treatment, and to begin to educate the patient about anxious-depressive distress and its physical and psychological effects. Culturally appropriate analogies promote the acceptance and recall of the core teaching principles. In this first session, the main metaphor utilized is that of the "inner child" who remembers everything and is easily frightened. This is used as a way to teach about bad memory triggers and about emotional hijacking.

In this session, meditation and applied stretching are introduced. The therapist should be sure that the patient does the stretching and other motions, and if the patient doesn't, encourage the patient to do so with a playful mien. The therapist should maintain a playful (even laughing) demeanor whenever possible. At times, to ensure that a sense of relaxation is being conveyed, the therapist should purposefully slow down and deepen the voice. This also creates a sense of shift in the session and so promotes flexibility and emotion regulation.

Outline of Session 1

- Core lessons

    1. Education about anxious-depressive distress (symptoms)
    2. Creating positive treatment expectancy
        ➢ Introduce treatment goals
        ➢ Create positive expectancy about the treatment through metaphors

    3. Education about anxious-depressive distress (the inner child metaphor)
    4. Emotion regulation techniques
        ➢ Teach about the effect of attentional focus on mood
        ➢ Emotion-distancing protocol: Mood awareness, labeling, and distancing
        ➢ Introducing multisensorial awareness

- Stretching module for before bed
    ○ Behind-the-back, straight-arm stretch
    ○ Above-the-head, straight-arm stretch

- Homework
    ○ Stretching before bed
    ○ Emotion-distancing protocol

- ○ Living in the moment
- ○ Week's meditation lesson

- Meditation upon returning home and during the coming week
  - ○ Leaf-movement awareness
  - ○ Mindful eating

Core Lesson 1: Education about Anxious-Depressive Distress

• Educating about Symptoms of Anxious-Depressive Distress and Modifying Catastrophic Cognitions about Them

Symptoms of anxious-depressive distress are not dangerous. This illness is not dangerous, but it does cause distress.

Symptoms of Anxious-Depressive Distress

Anxiety and depression may cause some of the following symptoms and problems:

- Constant recall of disturbing things that happened in the past
- Vivid recall of the past event as if it were happening again
- Startle, for example, feeling very anxious and distressed, even shocked, if you hear a sudden noise
- Panic, suddenly feeling afraid
- Various somatic symptoms such as the following:
  - ○ bodily tension
  - ○ neck soreness
  - ○ headache
  - ○ tinnitus
  - ○ shortness of breath
  - ○ palpitations
  - ○ dizziness

- Bodily symptoms that make you think you are going to have a heart attack, though there is really no danger
- Bodily symptoms that make you think you'll suffocate, though that is really not the case
- Bodily symptoms that make you think you have a major health problem, though you don't [here the therapist can mention certain cultural syndromes of the group in question that concern anxiety/distress]
- Irritability
- Poor concentration
- Worrying a lot; not being able to stop thinking about this or that problem
- Feeling as if your memory is going bad; that you will become crazy
- Poor sleep
- Nightmare
- Sleep paralysis

Normalizing the Symptoms of Anxious-Depressive Distress

These are common symptoms and problems for people experiencing anxious-depressive distress. There is no danger.

> "If I had experienced anxiety and depression, then I would have these symptoms, too."

Nothing Wrong with the Mind

These symptoms do not mean you are crazy. [It is important to stress that psychopathology is not tantamount to *madness*, as many Muslims living in Western cultures originate from countries that, for cultural reasons, tend to equate such psychopathology with madness (e.g., in Arabic referred to as "*majnoon*").]

Nothing Wrong with the Body

These symptoms from distress are not dangerous and will not harm you.

Improve with Treatment

All these symptoms will improve with treatment.

• Eliciting Patient Symptoms to Be Targeted in Treatment

Do you have any of the symptoms that I just described, like cold hands and feet, palpitations, or getting angry often?

Are there other symptoms that you want us to help with?

Which symptoms or problems are most troublesome? Please describe.

Core Lesson 2: Creating Positive Expectancy about Treatment

• Stating Treatment Goals

Goals: Decreased Symptoms and Increased Psychological and Emotional Flexibility

The treatment aims to help you in various ways. These include the following:

- *Reduce symptoms.* The aim of treatment is to reduce many of the symptoms you may experience, like your heart sometimes pounding in your chest, or getting angry.
- *Learn how to relax.* The goal is to teach you how to concentrate, to be able to live in the present moment, and to create positive emotions to calm the mind.
- *Learn to distance yourself from emotion.* When you have an emotion like anger, the treatment will help you distance yourself from that emotion, change to another mood, control your emotion, or not act on it.
- *Learn to relax your muscles and be flexible in your body.* In the treatment, you will learn how to relax your muscles and be more flexible in your body.
- *Learn to be more flexible in your thoughts and feelings.* In the treatment, you will learn how to be more emotionally and psychologically flexible, to be better at adjusting to problems and situations as they arise.

- *Learn not to think about the past so much.* In the treatment, you will learn to think about the past less, so you can resolve the problems you have now.
- *Learn to be a good model for others in your family.* The skills you learn, you can also teach others in your family, for example, your children.

• Create Positive Expectancy and Patience about the Treatment Process through Analogies

Length of Treatment: Ten Sessions

We will teach you something new each week. There are a total of ten sessions.

Stair Analogy

The treatment is like climbing the stairs. You must go up one stair at a time. [Here the therapist could mention verses from the Quran and sayings of prophet Muhammad, stressing the importance of being patient in order to achieve one's goals and that Allah loves those who are patient; e.g., the Quran says, "So be patient with gracious patience" (70:5); "be patient, and your patience is not but through Allah" (16:127); "Allah loves the patient ones" (3:146); "Oh you who believe, seek help through patience and prayer. Indeed, Allah is with those who are patient" (2:153); and the prophet Muhammad said, "whoever is patient Allah will bestow patience upon him, and no one is ever given anything better and more generous than patience" (as found in the *Sahih Al-Bukhari* collection).]

Food Analogy: Multiple Steps to Make a Special Food

The treatment is like making a special food dish. There are various steps needed and many ingredients, too. It is just like when you make . . . [here the therapist can describe a dish that involves several steps; the patient can be asked directly about a particular food in their culture. Muslims are rooted in a multiplicity of countries with unique food cultures and cuisines. For example, here the therapist could mention the food dish known as *biryani*, a very common dish in many majority Muslim countries. The therapist could mention that one first has to cook the rice, then add garlic paste, chopped onions, and tomatoes, then stir the dish until onions soften; then one adds vegetables of choice, such as chilies, coriander leaves, and carrots; one can fry chopped chicken in a different pan, and then add this to the dish as well, etc.]

Core Lesson 3: Education about Anxious-Depressive Distress: Inner Child Analogy

• The Inner Child (Translating the Concept of the Limbic System)

There is a part of us that recalls all the things that we have experienced, especially frightening things. This might be called an inner child.

• The Inner Child Remembers All, Especially Bad Things

The inner child keeps thinking of distressing events
- A scared inner child tells us over and over, "Watch out! Bad things could happen again!"

- Part of our brain is like a young child inside us who remembers all past bad things and is continually getting frightened or sad.
- The inner child wants to warn us. But it warns too much, even when there is no danger.
- When upset, the inner child will cause you to have strong emotions for no reason, such as feeling angry or sad, or symptoms such as having your heart beat fast.

The inner child remembers everything associated with the distress

This part of us, this scared inner child, has a very special function. Whenever a bad thing happens, the inner child remembers not only the bad thing that happened but also everything associated with the event. The inner child may remember the following about the bad event:

- Weather conditions
- Appearance of people
- Smells
- Sounds
- Somatic symptoms you had at that time, like dizziness or shortness of breath
- Mood, like fear

Things associated with the anxious-depressive distress cause the inner child to recall the distress

So now if anything occurs that also occurred during a distressing past event, the inner child thinks that bad things will happen. Some triggers of bad memories may be:

- *Weather conditions: Rainy day example.* If it is a rainy day, it may bring to mind a bad thing that happened on a rainy day.
- *Weather conditions: Overcast day.* If it is overcast, it may bring to mind a bad thing that happened on a cloudy day.
- *Appearance of persons.* If the person who hurt you was bald, when you see a bald person, it may bring to mind a bad thing the first bald person did to you.
- *Smells.* If you encounter a certain smell, it may bring to mind a bad thing that happened when you smelled that same smell.
- *Sound.* If you hear a loud sound, it may bring back feelings and images from the times you heard loud noises in the past, such as bombs blowing up or a door slamming when someone hurt you.
- *Somatic symptoms.* If you develop a headache, or pounding in your chest, it may bring to mind bad things that happened to you in the past, because you had those symptoms when bad things happened to you in the past.
- *Mood: Depression example.* When you are sad, it may bring to mind bad things that happened in the past that made you sad, or of all the times you were sad in the past.

• May Not Know That the Inner Child Has Been Reminded of the Past: Reframing Symptoms and Emotions as Caused by a Bad Memory

You may not be aware of what your inner child has noticed that reminds it of the past, causing you to feel irritable, scared, or sad. You may also have a pounding heart or shortness of breath, all because you have been unknowingly reminded of a past thing.

• Self-Soothing

If your inner child thinks of the past and is frightened or sad, do the following:

- *Soothe.* Tell the inner child not to be afraid.
- *Reassure.* Reassure this inner child that we are now here in [mention the country], in the city of [name the city], that you are no longer in [name the country or place where the distress occurred], and that there is no reason now to feel so afraid or sad.
- *Bring to the present.* If anything causes the inner child to think of the past, comfort the inner child by saying, "Don't worry, that was the past! Come into the present moment."
- *Comfort.* Comfort the inner child.
  - Rock it
  - Soothe it[1]
  - Sing to it

[Here the therapist can mention that the inner child may be soothed by doing *dhikr*; and that the *Quran* encourages us to call upon God using His different names (see Quran verse 17:110–111), and that he or she may evoke these names of Allah and ponder their deeper meanings to soothe the inner child. Those names of God that make the inner child feel safe should be used such as *ar-Rahman* (the Most Merciful), *al-Wadood* (the Most Loving), *al-Mumin* (the Granter of Security), *al-Muhaymin* (the Protector), *al-Gafur* (the Forgiving), *al-Salam* (the Ultimate Provider of Peace), *al-Muqit* (the Nourisher), and so on (see Table 2 for selected names of God, which may be handed out to the patient. The patient can also just ponder one or more of the names of Allah such as The Ever-Forgiving or The Most Loving [Table 2].) Another *dhikr* called *tasbeeh* that a patient may say to soothe the inner child is repeating each of three distinct praises of God – *subhanAllah* (glory be to God; thirty-three times), *alhamdulilah* (praise be to God; thirty-three times), *Allahuakbar* (God is the greatest; thirty-four times) – all the while using his or her fingers to count (*tasbeeh*). Also, one can mention to the patient the following verses in the Quran, in which God says, "in the remembrance of God the hearts find rest" (Quran: 13:28) and "Allah doesn't burden a soul beyond its capacity" (Quran 2:286), and one can give reassurance that the *dhikr* may bring inner peace and comfort to the inner child and that God tests us to make us stronger but never beyond what we are able to bear.[2]]

• What Causes Your Inner Child to be Afraid or Sad? Eliciting Anxious-Depressive Distress Triggers

What causes you to think of past bad things? Is it the weather, or something you see on TV that leads you to worry about things? Try to notice this in the next week.

---

[1] Some Muslim males (for cultural reasons, as it may go against established ideals of masculinity; for more details, see Introduction) might not be comfortable with soothing and rocking an inner child (this may be emasculating); in these cases, this analogy may require special framing. If the patient does not respond well to this analogy, the clinician should explain that the inner child simply refers to an inner part of himself. In some cases, one may simply recommend *dhikr*, as a type of inner soothing (instead of soothing the inner child).

[2] Note that religious examples should be used with caution. Some patients may not be religious in which case the religious rephrasing may be used as an example to make the concepts more understandable.

Core Lesson 4: Teaching Emotion Regulation Techniques

• Education: Attention Focus and Mood: The Fleeting Nature of Emotion

You should know that whatever you put your mind on will determine how you feel. If you put your mind on a good attentional object, your mood will improve.

- *Television example.* If you think of a problem, you may feel angry and upset. Then if you watch a TV program that you like, that feeling will go away. [If, in the culture, certain TV or online streaming shows (e.g., on YouTube) are popular, these should be mentioned, even a specific one.]
- *Religious example.* Or if you do a religious thing, this too may take your mind off worries and help your mood. [The following can be suggested, the patient choosing the method that appeals to him or her]:
  - Making *dhikr* (i.e., engaging in the remembrance of Allah), e.g., by evoking Allah's many names, such as The Ever-Forgiving and The Most Loving, and pondering their deeper meanings (see Table 2);
  - Making *dua* (i.e., supplicating), e.g., while evoking God's names and attributes and asking for forgiveness, and/or asking for help in worldly matters such as asking God to cure all illness and remove financial difficulties;
  - Doing *tasbeeh* (repeating each of three distinct praises of God thirty-three or thirty-four times as appropriate while using the fingers to count);
  - Doing *salah* (ritualistic prayer performed five times a day, involving standing, bowing, and prostrating, explained in the Introduction), done with complete attentional focus on God (e.g., on His infinite mercy and glory), called *kushoo*, which may entail spending prolonged time (e.g., several minutes) in the various physical postures (e.g., bowing or prostrating) [the therapist can mention that the prophet Muhammad would spend hours doing *salah*, e.g., prostrating for long periods];
  - Reciting the Quran;
  - Doing *ruqya,* which entails reciting Quranic verses and then gently blowing on various parts of one's body, or reciting verses over a bucket of water used for drinking or bathing, or even on olive oil (it is not uncommon to massage such olive oil on the body prior to sleep); and/or
  - Doing *wudhu* (ritualistic washing of the face, arms, and feet) [the therapist can remind the patient that during *wudhu* any body part that comes in contact with water is cleansed of sin; for instance, by rinsing the mouth it is cleansed from sins, such as profanities uttered during the course of the day; and the patient can be reminded that Muslims are encouraged to be mindful of God during *wudhu,* such as when water is running down the limbs to cleanse off sins.]

- *Going outside may help.* If you go out and do something, this will change your mood.

• Education and Practice of an Emotion Regulation Technique: Mood Awareness, Labeling, and Distancing

- *Mood awareness.* At this moment, and in the next week, try to notice your moods, such as anger or sadness; practice being aware of your moods.
- *Labeling emotion.* Observe your mood, and label it, such as anger, fear, worry, envy, hate, happiness, excitement.
- *Emotional distancing.* Just let the emotion go; just stay at a distance from it and watch it.
- *Cloud analogy for emotional distancing.* Know that any mood is like a cloud, which will soon pass away from your mind like a cloud moves from the sky. Just watch your mood, like a cloud in the sky. [The therapist should point out the window, at the sky, and if there is cloud, at the cloud.]

• Education and Practice of an Emotion Regulation Technique: Living in the Moment with All the Senses

Rationale for Living in the Moment with All the Senses (Mindfulness)

- *Relaxation.* Keeping your mind just on what is happening right now, around you, at this moment, will cause relaxation.
- *A good image in your mind.* Mood is determined by what you think about, what you attend to. The world, what is going on your senses, is always happening, and always there for you to pay attention to. It is a good attention object.

Living in the Moment with All the Senses: Staying with the Here and Now

- *Living in the now.* We want to teach you to try to be aware of the present moment, to bring all your senses to bear upon what is actually happening here and now.
- *Don't have you mind float to the past or future.* You do not want your mind to imagine what will happen in an hour, or to float to the past and what happened this morning or yesterday, or what occurred last week, a year ago, or long ago.
- *Live in the moment with all the senses.* You need to bring your mind to the moment, to be aware of all your senses, right now. [The therapist should slow the rate of speaking as he or she says the following, and should point to the part of the body related to the senses: to the eye, ear, nose]:
  - What you see
  - What you hear
  - What you smell
  - How the breath flows
  - How your arm feels as you move it through space [The therapist should bend the arm slowly, attending to how it feels.]

Practice Living in the Moment with All Your Senses When You Are Upset

When you become upset or scared, practice multisensorial living in the moment. Try the following:

- *Come into the moment: Time and place.* Try to be aware only of the present moment, here around you, right now, here in this country [mention the country], here in this city [mention the city], to what is around you right now, at this moment.
- *Come into the moment: The senses.* Try to be aware of what is going around you, with one or more your senses.
  - *Sounds.* Attend to sounds around you, such as the following [the therapist should point at the ear, and describe ambient sounds, pausing after the description of each type of sound, with the following being some examples]: The sound of –
    - cars going by, their engines, the tires moving along the street
    - people talking
    - the air conditioner
    - your own breathing

  - *Visual images.* Attend to sights around you, such as the following [if there is a window, the therapist should describe tree branches, leaves, outside the window]:
    - *Shapes.* The shape of –
      - leaves
      - clouds

    - *Colors.* The color of
      - leaves
      - clouds

      [The therapist should describe the color of objects outside the window, pausing a few seconds after describing each one; most objects have different colors, such as a leaf with its different shades of green, and those color variations in the object should be mentioned.]

    - *Motion.* The movement of –
      - branches and leaves in the wind, which may also make sounds

      [The therapist points at the object outside the window, describing the motion, however slight it might be.]

Week's Stretching Module with a Paired Instructional Metaphor

Introduction to Stretching

We want to teach you how to stretch. Each week we will teach you to stretch.

Handout of Stretching

All the stretches are in a handout with pictures to remind you how to do the stretching. Here it is. [Give this to the patient; see Appendix A.]

Rationale for Stretching

Help Sleep

It will help you to sleep because it

- ○ will help you relax
- ○ will prevent cramps

Flexible Body, Flexible Mind

If you are more relaxed and flexible in your body, it will help you to be more relaxed and more flexible in your emotions, mind, and ways of thinking.

Help Make You Feel Better When Upset

If you stretch when you are upset, it will make you feel better.

Embodying Metaphors

While doing the stretching, think of the following [the therapist should repeat this self-statement while the actual stretching is being done]:

➤ "As I become more flexible in my body, may I become more flexible in my thoughts, in my emotions, may I know how to adjust to each new situation." [The therapist can mention here that this may also be done as a *dua* (i.e., a supplication); e.g., "Oh Allah, may I become more flexible in my body, may I become more flexible in my thoughts, in my emotions, may I know how to adjust to each new situation."]

Relaxing the Shoulders: Behind-the-Back, Straight-Arm Stretch[3]

1. Stand.
2. Put your arms behind your back.
3. Clasp your hands together, fingers interlocking.
4. Straighten your arms.
5. Keeping your arms straight, and your hands clasped, raise your arms until you feel a little tension.
6. Hold your arms there and count to ten slowly.
7. Unclasp your hands, and let your arms fall to your side.
8. Repeat one or two more times if desired.

Relaxing the Shoulders: Above-the-Head, Straight-Arm Stretch

1. Stand.
2. Put your arms straight ahead and clasp your hands together, fingers interlocking.
3. Straighten your arms, producing a little tension, all the while keeping your hands clasped together.
4. Keeping your arms straight and your hands clasped together, make an upward arc by raising them upwards above your head.
5. Reach up as far as you can so that you straighten your body and spine and arms, creating a pulling feeling.

---

[3] For this and the following stretches, the therapist models how to do the stretching and the patient imitates. The therapist should discretely observe the patient, to make sure it is done appropriately. If correction is needed, make sure to complement the patient, and to smile, when making corrections.

6. Keeping your arms straight and your hands clasped together, bend from one side to another, slowly, feeling the pulling tension in your arms.
7. Do this two or three times, one side and then another, all the while making sure to pull up, to reach as high as possible.
8. Unclasp your hands, and let your arms fall to your side.
9. Repeat one or two more times if desired.

When to Practice Stretching
You should practice these stretches at the following times:

Practice Stretching upon Returning Home
When you get home, practice the stretching we taught you today. Do each stretch three times.

Practice Stretching Every Night before Bed
Every night, before you go to bed, for example when you are watching television, practice the stretches we have taught you.

Practice Stretching when You Are Upset
If you practice stretching when you are upset, it will make you feel better. [Here the therapist could mention that *salah* may also be performed to feel better, such as at the various times during the day in the time windows specified in the Islamic faith (e.g., before going to bed) or when feeling upset; could mention that the patient may remain in the various physical postures (e.g., bowing and prostrating) for an extended period (e.g., several seconds to minutes), which also stretches the body to make it more flexible and relaxed.]

Homework
Stretching before Sleep
Practice the stretch we taught you today, in particular before going to bed. Use the handout to guide you while doing the stretches. You can do the stretches while watching television before bed. [And you can do *salah* to improve bodily flexibility.]

Practice Labeling Emotions and Detached and Curious Observation
This week, practice the following:

- *Notice your emotion.* Be aware of your emotions.
- *Label your emotion.* Observe your mood, and label it, whether the emotion is anger, fear, worry, disgust, anxiety, happiness, excitement, etc.
- *Cloud analogy.* Watch your thoughts and moods like you would observe clouds passing across the sky.
- *Detached and curious observation.* Just watch your mood, not acting on it, looking at it like a cloud in the sky, which will soon pass away. Observe your moods with a detached and curious observation and distance yourself from your emotion, observing it.

Living in the Moment with All Your Senses

As you go home, we want you to practice living in the moment and attending to your senses (i.e., mindfulness) and to what is around you right now. Practice this in the following week.

To Practice Upon Leaving the Office: Meditation Lesson

The Attention Object Determines Mood: Finding Good Objects

What you put your mind on will determine your mood, how you feel. Put your mind on a good object, on something that will improve your mood.[4] [Here the therapist can mention: (1) making *dhikr* (i.e., engaging in the remembrance of Allah), e.g., by evoking one or more of Allah's many names such as The Ever-Forgiving or The Most Loving (Table 2) and pondering their deeper meanings; (2) making *dua* (i.e., supplicating, e.g., while evoking God's names and attributes and asking for forgiveness, and/or asking for help in worldly matters); (3) doing *tasbeeh* (repeating thirty-three times each of three distinct praises of God while using the fingers to count); (4) doing *salah* (ritualistic prayer), done with complete attentional focus on God (i.e., *kushoo*); (5) reciting the Quran; (6) doing *ruqyah*, e.g., by reciting Quranic verses and then gently blowing on various parts of your own body, or over a bucket of water to drink or bath in, or even over olive oil to massage on the body; and (7) doing *wudhu* (ritualistic washing of the face, arms, and feet), while mindful of water running down the limbs and cleansing off sins.]

Explanation for Practicing Present-Moment Awareness (Mindfulness)

- *Keeping your mind on a good object.* Paying attention to what is going on around you as you go home or to what is going on around you right now, such as sounds, colors, movements, will keep your mind on a good thing.
- *Prevent your mind from floating to the past, floating to the future.* By paying attention to something going on around you right now, your mind will not float to the past or to the future, to upsetting thoughts and concerns.
- *Don't miss the beauty around you.* Often as we walk along, we think of various problems or feel angry towards something or someone, and we forget to look at the beauty of what is around us. We are thinking about this or that, feeling angry about something, are in our heads, and we walk by something beautiful, say a beautiful tree, beautiful colored leaves, and don't even notice it. We are in our heads, in our thoughts, in our anger, and fail to notice what is going on around us. [A way to promote such sensorial awareness is by asking patients to contemplate the beauty of God's creation such as clouds, trees, and how the leaves move with the wind. One can mention to the patient that the Quran stresses in several verses the importance of noticing the beautiful creation of God: for example, "this is the creation of God. So show Me what those other than Him have created" (31:11); "[such is] the artistry of God [i.e., referring to the creation], who perfected all things" (27:88); "[God]perfected everything which He created" (32:7).]

---

[4] When teaching the meditation method, the therapist should make sure that his or her voice slows, and possibly deepens, in order to promote a sense of relaxation. The therapist should feel relaxed; the therapist should slow down the pace to the point that he or she feels relaxed.

Leaf-Movement Mindfulness (Or Leaf-and-Branch-Movement Mindfulness)[5]

On your way home today, we want you just to watch how the wind moves the leaves and branches. Watch how the leaves and branches dance, moving slightly in the wind, how they rise, and fall. [The therapist should point out the window at an example. If there are no leaves, instruct the patient to notice how the branches bob in the wind.]

Mindful Eating

When you are home today pay special attention to the foods you eat. Pay full attention to their rich flavors, smells, and textures with all your senses. [Here the therapist can mention that the prophet Muhammad said that "when one of you eats some food, let him say *Bismillah* (i.e., in the name of God),"[6] and also taught his followers to praise Allah upon finishing eating: for instance, "Allah is pleased with His servant [or slave] when he eats something and praises Him for it, or drinks something and praises Him for it."[7] The therapist can also mention that the Prophet stressed the importance of not overeating (e.g., he said, "a man does not fill any vessel worse than his stomach.")[8] The therapist may remind the patient of the overall benefits of not overeating (e.g., energy, weight loss, and reduced bodily inflammation). The therapist can mention occasional fasting (e.g., one or two times a week) as an option (i.e., if the patient is otherwise healthy and accustomed to fasting during *ramadhan*); mention that the Prophet, in addition to the month of *ramadhan*, used to fast Monday and Thursday,[9] and that such fasting makes the body lighter and reduces laziness. It also makes one more grateful for food (i.e., upon breaking the fast). Mention that the patient should pay special attention to (i.e., fully concentrate on) the fast-breaking foods with all the senses (e.g., flavours, smells, and textures).]

---

[5] This is taking the leaf as the object of attention. This is leaf mindfulness, a form of multisensorial living in the present, because if the patient takes the leaf as an object of concentration, the patient is also attending to something occurring around him or her in the present moment.

[6] Narration found in the at-Tirmidhi collection.

[7] Found in the Muslim collection.

[8] Narration found in the at-Tirmidhi collection.   [9] Narration found in the at-Tirmidhi collection.

Applied Stretching and the Toe-to-Head Muscle Relaxation with Visualization

Overview of Core Lessons

"Applied muscle relaxation" is traditionally used to describe the relaxation of muscles by contracting a muscle, holding the contraction, and then releasing tension. This might also be called contract-release muscle relaxation. Another method of muscle relaxation, such as that used in yoga, involves stretching a muscle by forced elongation, holding the forced elongation a certain time, and then releasing it. This might also be called elongation-release relaxation or stretch-release relaxation. Multiplex CBT teaches both applied muscle relaxation (i.e., contract-release relaxation) and applied muscle stretching (i.e., elongation-release relaxation).[1]

Patients who experience anxious-depressive distress have multiple symptoms induced by muscle tension. Examples of sensations caused by muscle tension include joint soreness, muscle soreness, and headache. In addition, those muscle-tension-caused somatic sensations often give rise to catastrophic cognitions, trigger distress associations, and activate interceptive conditioning. In addition, muscle relaxation will decrease arousal and hence fear, and this reduced arousal and fear will decrease symptoms such as cold extremities. Furthermore, applied muscle stretching allows for the introduction of phrases and images that promote a positive self-image of flexibility and prime to being flexible. These are embodied metaphors.

The therapist should be sure that the patient does the stretching and other motions, and if the patient does not, the therapist should encourage the patient to do so, all the while with a playful mien, a playful demeanor; this models a positive way of interacting and it also creates new positive associations to the topics being discussed. At times, to promote relaxation, the therapist should purposefully slow and deepen the voice. This also creates a sense of shift in the session: a shift in voice and emotional register.

Outline of Session 2

- Homework review
- Core lessons
  1. Introducing applied muscle stretching
  2. Explaining the importance of applied muscle stretching
  3. Teach toe-to-head muscle relaxation with visualization

---

[1] In truth, both these methods achieve relaxation of tension in muscles and both achieve stretching, but approach the problem in different ways.

- Stretching module for before bed
  - Behind-the-back, straight-arm stretch
  - Above-the-head, straight-arm stretch
  - Shoulder roll stretch

- Homework
  - Stretching before sleep
  - Muscle tension awareness and applied muscle stretching
  - Week's meditation lesson

- Meditation upon returning home and during the coming week
  - Leaf movement
  - Leaf-and-color mindfulness
  - Leaf-movement mindfulness paired with a flexibility metaphor
  - Mindful eating

Homework Review

• Living in the Moment upon Returning Home

As you went home at the end of the last session, and during the last week, did you practice living in the moment, paying attention to how leaves and branches moved in the wind?

• Stretching before Sleep

Last week did you practice stretching each night before going to sleep? Do you have the sheet showing the stretches, or do you need a new one?

Core Lesson 1: Applied Muscle Stretching (AMS)

• Using Applied Muscle Stretching to Prevent Symptoms

Practice relaxing muscles in order to prevent getting anxious or depressed, OR getting headaches and other symptoms. It will also help you to feel more psychologically and emotionally flexible. You can do it as you wait for a doctor, or at other times.

• Relaxing Areas of Tension: Arm Rotation with Wrist Rotation

Let us use an arm example, but you can stretch however you want, wherever you feel tense. Watch me and do the following:[2]
1. Straight-arm rotational stretching
   i. Straighten the arms until slightly tense.
   ii. Rotate the straightened arms, once in one direction, then in the other.
   iii. Repeat as desired with one or two arms.

---

[2] The therapist needs to model these actions, doing what he or she instructs the patient to do, providing a model. The aim is to stretch and relax all the joints in the arm, including the shoulder joint, elbow, wrist, and fingers.

2. Bent-arm rotational stretching.
    i. Bend one arm a little, however much you want.
    ii. Rotate at the wrist several times.
    iii. Repeat as desired.
3. Finger stretch
    i. Straighten out the fingers of one hand until there is some tension.
    ii. Wiggle the fingers.
    iii. Repeat as desired.
4. Repeat any of the above as desired. [The therapist repeats any of the above stretches.]

• Stretch However It Feels Good

Do any movements that relax the body. [The therapist can model any stretching at this point, as in rotating the head, opening the mouth, then making side-to-side motions.]

• Embodying Flexibility Metaphors

While doing the stretching, think of the following [the therapist should repeat this self-statement while the actual stretching is being done]:

➤ "As I become more flexible in my body, may I become more flexible in my thoughts, in my emotions, may I know how to adjust to each new situation." [Or, "Oh Allah may I become more flexible in my body, may I become more flexible in my thoughts, in my emotions, may I know how to adjust to each new situation."]

Core Lesson 2: Explaining Why Muscle Relaxation is Important

• How Muscle Tension Results

If you worry about your problems, if you are afraid, soon you will increase muscle tension in your body.

• Somatic Symptoms and Mood Symptoms Caused by Muscle Tension

Body Symptoms Caused by Muscle Tension

If your muscles are tight, such as muscles in your arms, legs, neck, and head, it may cause many symptoms, including the following:

➤ headache
➤ neck soreness
➤ sore arms and legs
➤ arm numbness
➤ cold arms and hands
➤ trembling in the arms, hands, and legs

Mood Symptoms Caused by Muscle Tension

If you are tight in the body, it will cause you to feel anxious, to feel tense.

• Modifying Catastrophic Cognition about Muscle-Tension-Caused Somatic Symptoms

Addressing Catastrophic Cognitions: General Reframing

When you get these symptoms, realize they are from muscle tension, not from a dangerous problem with your body. Do not fear symptoms like cold hands and feet, like neck tension and soreness, or shakiness of the arms and hands. These symptoms are just from muscle tension and distress.

Addressing Catastrophic Cognitions: Addressing Fears of Potential Cultural Syndromes and Ethnophysiological Disturbance

These symptoms do not indicate any disturbance of the body, and they are not dangerous. They do not indicate any problem with your body.

• Why We Want to Teach You Muscle Relaxation and Stretching

Relaxed Body, Relaxed Mind

We want you to learn how to relax your muscles so you can relax your mind.

Flexible Body, Flexible Mind

We want you to learn to stretch your muscles so you will be more flexible in your thinking and emotions.

Decrease Muscle-Tension-Caused Symptoms

We want you to learn how to relax your muscles so you will relax, so you will:
- not be so tense
- not get so sore or cold in your arms and legs
- not get so sore in the neck
- not get so many headaches
- not be so shaky in your arms and legs

• Muscle Relaxation and Muscle Mindfulness

Learning to Recognize When You Are Tight in the Body

You will learn to recognize when you are becoming tense.

Muscle-Tension Awareness as Part of Living in the Moment with All Your Senses

Being aware of tension in your body is another part of learning to live in the present moment.

Relax Any Areas of Tension

Stretch and relax any areas of tension you notice. We will teach you many ways to do this.

Core Lesson 3: Teaching Toe-to-Head Relaxation with Visualization

Now we want to teach you a way to make yourself feel better in your body and mind to be more flexible in your body and mind:

➡***Go to Appendix B and do the Toe-to-Head Relaxation with Visualization***

Week's Stretching Module with a Paired Instructional Metaphor

• Introduction

We want to teach you how to stretch. Each week we will teach you to stretch.

Handout

Handout of Stretches

All the stretches are in a handout with pictures to remind you how to do the stretching. Do you still have that handout? [If not, give to the patient]

• Rationale for Stretching

Help Sleep

It will help you to sleep because it
○ will help you relax
○ will prevent cramps

Flexible Body, Flexible Mind

If you are more relaxed and flexible in your body, it will help you to be more relaxed and more flexible in your emotions, mind, and ways of thinking.

Help Making You Feel Better When Upset

If you stretch when you are upset, it will make you feel better.

• Embodying Metaphors

While doing the stretching, think of the following [the therapist should repeat this self-statement while the actual stretching is being done]:

➢ "As I become more flexible in my body, may I become more flexible in my thoughts, in my emotions, may I know how to adjust to each new situation." [Or, "Oh Allah may I become more flexible in my body, may I become more flexible in my thoughts, in my emotions, may I know how to adjust to each new situation."]

• Relaxing the Shoulders: Behind-the-Back, Straight-Arm Stretch

1. Stand.

2. Put the arms behind your back.
3. Grasp the hands together, the fingers interlocking.
4. Straighten the arms.
5. Keeping the arms straight, and the hands clasped, raise the arms until you feel a little tension.
6. Hold the arms there and count to ten slowly.
7. Unclasp the hands, and let the arms fall to your side.
8. Repeat one or two more times if desired.

• Relaxing the Shoulders: Above-the-Head, Straight-Arm Stretch

1. Stand.
2. Put your two arms forward and straight ahead and then grasp the hands together, the fingers interlocking.
3. Straighten the arms, producing a little tension, all the while keeping the hands clasped together.
4. Keeping the arms straight and the hands clasped together, make an upward arc by raising them upwards above the head.
5. Reach up as far as you can so that you straighten your body and spine and arms, creating a pulling feeling.
6. Keeping the arms straight and the hands clasped together, bend from one side to another, slowly, feeling the pulling tension in the arms.
7. Do this two or three times, one side and then another, all the while making sure to pull up, to reach as high as possible.
8. Unclasp the hands, and let the arms fall to your side.
9. Repeat one or two more times if desired.

• Relaxing the Shoulders: Rolling-the-Shoulders Stretch

1. Stand.
2. Roll the shoulders forward.
3. Roll the shoulders back.
4. Roll the shoulders forward.
5. Roll the shoulders back.
6. Try to tighten the stomach muscles a little as you do it.
7. Repeat one or two more times if desired.

• Arm Relaxation: Straight-Arm Rotation Method

1. *Straighten both arms straight ahead and bend wrists.* Straighten both arms completely straight while bending the wrists, and feel the sense of stretching.
2. *Rotate the straightened arms in one direction.* Rotate the straightened arms until you feel slight tension.
3. *Rotate the straightened arms in the other direction.* Rotate the straightened arms in the other direction until you feel slight tension and hold them there a few seconds.

4. *Rotate the arms back-and-forth, with the wrists bent back and fingers straightened.* With the wrists back and the fingers straightened, rotate the arms back-and-forth, feeling the sense of tension.
5. When you are tense, you can stretch both arms, or one arm, in this way [The therapist should model the stretch with one arm.]
6. Repeat one or two more times if desired.

• When to Practice Stretching

You should practice these stretches at the following times:

Practice upon Returning Home

When you go home today you should practice this, so you will not forget.

Practice before Bed

You should also practice each night before going to bed, for instance, while watching television.

Practice Stretching When You Are Upset

If you do it when you are upset, it will make you feel better. [Here could mention that *salah* may also be performed to feel better, such as at the various times during the day in the time windows specified in the Islamic faith (e.g., before going to bed) or when feeling upset; could mention that the patient may remain in the various physical postures (e.g., bowing and prostrating) for an extended period (e.g., several seconds to minutes), which also stretches the body to make it more flexible and relaxed.]

Homework

Stretching before Sleep

Practice the stretch we taught you today, in particular before going to bed. Use the handout to guide you while doing the stretches.

You can do the stretches while watching television before bed. [And you can do *salah* to improve bodily flexibility.]

• Muscle Tension Awareness and Applied Muscle Stretching

During the day, try to be aware of the tension in your body, and stretch any area of tightness.
➤ Relax the shoulders
   ○ Stretch the shoulders by rolling them. [If the therapist notes an area of tightness in the patient, this should be stretched. The therapist can stretch any body area where he or she feels tight, because this tightness comes from sensing tightness in the patient.]

• Meditation Homework

As you go home, we want you to practice the following: practice putting your mind on a good thing, and practice this in the following week. It is also a way to practice living in the moment with all your senses.

To Practice Upon Leaving the Office: Meditation Lesson

• How the Attentional Object Determines Mood[3]

What you put your mind on will determine your mood, how you feel. Put your mind on a good object, on something that will improve your mood. For example, the Muslim religion teaches many ways to put the mind on God to enter a better state. [Here the therapist can mention: (1) *dhikr* (i.e., engaging in the remembrance of Allah), e.g., through recalling Allah's names such as The Ever Forgiving and The Most Loving; (2) *dua* (i.e., supplicating); (3) *tasbeeh* (repeating thirty-three or thirty-four times as appropriate each of three distinct praises of God while using the fingers to count; (4) *salah* (ritualistic prayer), done with complete attentional focus on God (i.e., *kushoo*); (5) reciting the Quran; (6) doing *ruqyah,* e.g., by reciting Quranic verses and then gently blowing on various parts of his/her own body; and (7) doing *wudhu* (ritualistic washing) while mindful of water running down the limbs and cleansing off sins.]

• Explanation for Practicing Present-Moment Awareness (Mindfulness)

Keeping your mind on a good object. Paying attention to what is going on around you as you go home, to what is going on around you right now, such as sounds, colors, movements, will keep your mind on a good thing.

Prevent your mind from floating to the past, floating to the future. By paying attention to something going on around you right now, your mind will not float to the past, to the future, to upsetting thoughts and concerns.

Don't miss the beauty around you. Often we walk along, we think of this problem or that, feel angry towards something or someone, and we forget to look at the beauty of what is around us. We are thinking about this or that, feeling angry about something, are in our heads, and we walk by something beautiful, say a beautiful tree or beautifully colored leaves, and don't even notice it. We are in our heads, in our thoughts, in our anger, and fail to notice what is going on around us. [A way to promote such sensorial awareness is by asking patients to contemplate the beauty of God's creation such as clouds, trees, and how the leaves move with the wind.]

• Leaf Mindfulness

On your way home today, we want you just to notice:

Leaf Movement

Notice the way the leaves and branches move in the wind. Watch how they dance in the wind. Note the way they rise and fall. [The therapist should point out the window at an example. If there are no leaves, branches can be focused on, or clouds.]

Leaf Shape and Color

Notice the shape of leaves, notice the color of leaves, and notice the play of light and shadow on the leaves.

---

[3] Remember to maintain a relaxed mood when teaching meditation, slowing down and deepening the voice to create a sense of relaxation.

Wind-moved Leaves and Branches as Teaching a Lesson, as Self-image (Metaphor): Flexibility Lesson[4]

As you watch the leaves moving in the wind, or the branches, ask that you can flexibly adjust to each new situation, just as the leaf (or branch) adjusts to each new current of wind.

• Mindful Eating

When you are home today pay special attention to the foods you eat. Pay full attention to their rich flavors, smells, and textures with all your senses. [Here the therapist can mention that the prophet Muhammad said, "when one of you eats some food, let him say *Bismillah* (i.e., in the name of God)," and also taught his followers to praise Allah upon finishing eating; for instance, "Allah is pleased with His servant when he eats something and praises Him for it, or drinks something and praises Him for it." Can also mention that the Prophet stressed the importance of not overeating; e.g., he said, "a man does not fill any vessel worse than his stomach." The therapist may remind the patient of the overall benefits of not overeating (e.g., energy, weight loss, and reduced bodily inflammation). The therapist can mention occasional fasting (e.g., one to two times a week) as an option (i.e., if the patient is otherwise healthy and accustomed to fasting during *ramadhan*); mention that the Prophet, in addition to the month of *ramadhan,* used to fast every Monday and Thursday, and that such fasting makes the body lighter and reduces laziness. It also makes one more grateful for food (i.e., upon breaking the fast). Mention that the patient should pay special attention to (i.e., fully concentrate on) the fast-breaking foods with all the senses (e.g., their flavors, smells, and textures).]

---

[4] Note that the patient is taught flexibility through multiple modalities. Through looking at the leaves moving in the wind, a nature exemplar of flexibility; by verbal reminders to be flexible; by switching sensory modalities. This is the multimodal teaching of psychological flexibility.

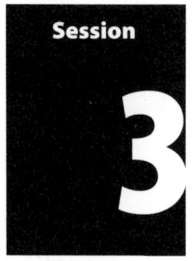

Session

3

Review of Toe-to-Head Muscle Relaxation with Visualization and the Introduction of the Dysphoria (Anxiety/Depression) Protocol, Education about Anxious-Depressive Distress and Teaching the Bad Memory Protocol (Emotion Regulation Toolbox)

Overview of Core Lessons

In this session, applied stretching is taught, and the patient is led once more through the whole body muscle relaxation (with contract-release and stretch-release relaxation) with visualization. As in almost all lessons, there is a section on mindfulness and stretching.

The chapter introduces a Bad Memory Protocol, which consists of a set of "tools," for example, emotion regulation and relaxation-type techniques, to be used when unwanted bad memories occur or when upset for any reason. It serves as practice in emotion regulation, being a set of emotion regulation techniques.

As indicated in the last session, the therapist should be sure that the patient does the stretching and other motions, and if the patient does not, the therapist should encourage the patient to do so, all the while with a playful mien, a playful demeanor. This models a positive way of interacting and it also creates new positive associations to the topics being discussed. At times, to promote relaxation, the therapist should purposefully slow and deepen the voice. This also creates a sense of shift in the session: a shift in voice and emotional register.

Outline of Session 3

- Homework review
- Core lessons
  1. Review the toe-to-head relaxation with visualization
  2. Review the applied muscle stretching
  3. Teach the dysphoria (anxiety/depression) protocol (an abbreviated form of the toe-to-head relaxation with visualization)

41

4. Education about bad memory
5. Teaching the bad memory protocol (emotion regulation toolbox)
- Stretching module for before bed
    - Behind-the-back, straight-arm stretch
    - Above-the-head, straight-arm stretch
    - Shoulder roll stretch
    - Straight-arm rotation stretch
- Homework
    - Stretching before sleep
    - Muscle tension awareness and applied stretching
    - Attending to candle imagery as flexibility primer
    - Week's meditation lesson
- Meditation upon returning home and during the coming week
    - Loving kindness

Homework Review

Living in the Moment upon Returning Home

As you went home at the end of the last session, and during the last week, did you practice living in the moment, paying attention to how leaves and branches moved in the wind?

Stretching before Sleep

Last week did you practice stretching each night before going to sleep? Do you have the sheet showing the stretches, or do you need a new one?

Core Lesson 1: Review of Toe-to-Head Relaxation with Visualization

Now we want to teach you a way to make yourself feel better in your body and mind, to be more flexible in your body and mind:

➤***Go to Appendix B and do the Toe-to-Head Relaxation with Visualization***

Core Lesson 2: Teaching Applied Muscle Relaxation (AMR) and Applied Muscle Stretching (AMS)

• Negative Consequences of Muscle Tension

You need to learn to be aware of when muscle tension builds up, and how to relax the tension. If not, the following may occur:

- *Somatic symptoms.* You will get headache, neck soreness, pain in the joints, and muscle cramps, and other symptoms, like cold hands and feet.

- *Anxious.* You will feel anxious and irritable.
- *Recall the past.* The tension and soreness and other somatic symptoms may cause you to think of past bad things.

• Addressing Catastrophic Cognitions

You need to learn to be aware of when muscle tension builds up, because it causes these symptoms, which are not dangerous, but they are bothersome.

• Treating Muscle Tension and Limb Coldness

You can treat muscle tension and cold extremities if it occurs by practicing how to relax and stretch muscles.

• Applied Muscle Stretching

Relax Any Tense Area

You should relax and stretch any area of identified tension. For example, you can [the therapist models]:

➢ Open the mouth wide and stretch it, moving it from side to side
➢ Massage your jaw

Washing Dishes and Chopping Ingredients Examples

While washing dishes or chopping dinner ingredients, or at other times, you may notice shoulder tension. Then you may want to relax the shoulders by doing the following [the therapist models]:

➢ Relaxing the shoulders
  1. Lightly lift up the shoulders and keep them up as you count to three.
  2. Let the shoulders drop.
  3. Roll the shoulders.
  4. Repeat one or two more times if needed.

Waiting in the Office Example

If you are waiting somewhere, like sitting in a waiting room for a long time, you can stretch any muscles that seem tense. You can do this with your legs, your arms, or neck.

Arm rotation protocol. Let us use an arm example.

[The therapist needs to model these actions, doing what he or she instructs the patient to do, providing a model. The aim is to stretch and relax all the joints in the arm, including the shoulder joint, elbow, wrist, and fingers. The therapist should be aware of making motions at those joints, either sequentially or simultaneously, as described below.]

1. Straight-arm rotational stretching
   i. Straighten the arms until slightly tense.
   ii. Rotate the straightened arms, once in one direction, then in the other.
   iii. Repeat as desired with one or two arms.

2. Bent-arm rotational stretching
    i. Bend one arm a little, however much you want.
    ii. Rotate at the wrist several times.
    iii. Repeat as desired.

3. Finger stretch
    i. Straighten out, and even arch, the fingers of one hand.
    ii. Wriggle the fingers.
    iii. Repeat as desired.

4. *Now stretch any area of tension* [The therapist should model this by moving the shoulders, stretching that area, or by stretching the mouth.]
5. *Applied stretching.* When you are tense, you can stretch one or both arms in this way. [The therapist should model the stretch with one arm.]

Embodying Flexibility Metaphors

While doing the stretching, think of the following [the therapist should repeat this self-statement while the actual stretching is being done]:

➤ "As I become more flexible in my body, may I become more flexible in my thoughts, in my emotions, may I know how to adjust to each new situation." [Or, "Oh Allah may I become more flexible in my body, may I become more flexible in my thoughts, in my emotions, may I know how to adjust to each new situation."]

Core Lesson 3: Teach the Dysphoria (Anxiety/Depression) Protocol[1]

• Eliciting Recent Distress Episode

In the last week, did you feel anxious or depressed for any reason? If so, why? [Ask just enough to get some sense of how the patient feels during the episodes.]

• Dysphoria (Anxiety/Depression) Protocol

If you are anxious or depressed, you can do any of the following to feel better:

—————————➤***Go to Appendix C and do the Dysphoria (Anxiety/Depression) Protocol***

---

[1] Please note that the anxiety/depression protocol is an abbreviated form of the toe-to-head muscle relaxation with visualization, focusing on the visualization part. It is AMR and AMS of the shoulders with the visualization and enactment of the visualized image.

Core Lesson 4: Education about Bad Memories

• Normalizing Bad Memories

As a result of anxious-depressive distress, it is normal that past events may return to your mind, sometimes like a film, like reliving the event, causing you to feel terrified again. It may seem as if the event is happening again, like you are back in that time again.

This is normal. You are not going crazy.

• Normalizing the Mind and Somatic Symptoms Associated with Bad Memories

Somatic Symptoms Associated with Bad Memories

When you think of the past, it may make you have many symptoms, like racing thoughts, a racing heart, shortness of breath, ringing in your ears, dizziness, or cold hands and feet.

Catastrophic Cognitions about the Induced Somatic Symptoms

You may fear something is wrong with your mind or body.

Modifying Catastrophic Cognitions

You are fine. Do not worry about something being wrong with your mind or body. Those symptoms are caused by distress, and will not harm you.

• Normalizing Bad Memories and Its Somatic Symptoms: The "I Too" Example

If I had gone through what you did, I would keep seeing those past memories, just like you, and would have the same symptoms.

Core Lesson 5: Teaching the Bad Memory Protocol (The Emotion Regulation Toolbox)

• Explore Recent Bad Memories

Presence of Bad Memories

In the last week, did you have any recall of the past when you didn't want to, either when awake or during a nightmare? If so, please describe.[2] [If the patient had no bad memories in the last week, then ask about the most recent episode, or about any upsetting event.]

---

[2] Through this, and the following questions, the goal is to have the patient, or a member of the group, share some bad memories. If a patient admits to having bad memories, and becomes visibly upset, the patient should be told not to recount the distressing event at this moment, and should also be told that the following can be used when he or she has bad memories. At that point, one should begin the Bad Memory Protocol (Emotion Regulation Toolbox) in Appendix D.

Presence of Flashback

Was your recall vivid, as if it were happening again? If so, please describe.

• Elicitation of Self-Treatment of a Bad Memory

When you had the bad memories, did you do anything to feel better?

• Bad Memory Protocol (Emotion Regulation Toolbox)[3]

When you have bad memories, or feel distressed, you can do any of the following. These are some tools you can use. Use whichever part you want to use.

➤***Go to Appendix D and do the Bad Memory Protocol (Emotion Regulation Toolbox)***

Week's Stretching Module with a Paired Instructional Metaphor

• Introduction

We want to teach you how to stretch. Each week we will teach you to stretch.

• Handout of Stretching

Handout of Stretches

All the stretches are in a handout with pictures to remind you how to do the stretching. Do you still have that handout? [If not, give to the patient.]

• Rationale for Stretching

Help Sleep

It will help you to sleep because it
○   will help you relax
○   will prevent cramps

Flexible Body, Flexible Mind

If you are more relaxed and flexible in your body, it will help you to be more relaxed and more flexible in your emotions, mind, and ways of thinking.

Help Make You Feel Better When Upset

If you stretch when upset, it will make you feel better.

---

[3]   The Bad Memory Protocol is a set of tools to be used when having bad memories. It is used in the treatment following elicitation of bad memories to promote emotional processing following elicitation of a distressing event. More broadly, the techniques can be used whenever distressed. Of note, doing the Bad Memory Protocol creates a sense of agency, a positive self-image of positive coping and flexibility, and it creates a new associate network to the distressing event.

• Embodying Metaphors

While doing the stretching, think the following [the therapist should ideally state this while the stretching is being done]:

➤ "As I become more flexible in my body, may I become more flexible in my thoughts, in my emotions, may I know how to adjust to each new situation." [Or, "Oh Allah may I become more flexible in my body, may I become more flexible in my thoughts, in my emotions, may I know how to adjust to each new situation."]

• Relaxing the Shoulders: Behind-the-Back, Straight-Arm Stretch

1. Stand.
2. Put the arms behind your back.
3. Grasp the hands together, the fingers interlocking.
4. Straighten the arms.
5. Keeping the arms straight, and the hands clasped, raise the arms until you feel a little tension.
6. Hold the arms there and count to ten slowly.
7. Unclasp the hands, and let the arms fall to your side.
8. Repeat one or two more times if desired.

• Relaxing the Shoulders: Above-the-Head, Straight-Arm Stretch

1. Stand.
2. Put your two arms forward and straight ahead and then grasp the hands together, the fingers interlocking.
3. Straighten the arms, producing a little tension, all the while keeping the hands clasped together.
4. Keeping the arms straight and the hands clasped together, make an upward arc by raising them upwards above the head.
5. Reach up as far as you can so that you straighten your body and spine and arms, creating a pulling feeling.
6. Keeping the arms straight and the hands clasped together, bend from one side to another, slowly, feeling the pulling tension in the arms.
7. Do this two or three times, one side and then another, all the while making sure to pull up, to reach as high as possible.
8. Unclasp the hands, and let the arms fall to your side.
9. Repeat one or two more times if desired.

• Relaxing the Shoulders: Rolling-the-Shoulders Stretch

1. Stand.
2. Roll the shoulders forward.
3. Roll the shoulders back.
4. Roll the shoulders forward.
5. Roll the shoulders back.
6. Try to tighten the stomach muscles a little as you do it.
7. Repeat one or two more times if desired.

• Arm Relaxation: Straight-Arm Rotation Method

1. *Straighten both arms straight ahead and bend wrists.* Straighten both arms completely straight while bending the wrists, and feel the sense of stretching.
2. *Rotate the straightened arms in one direction.* Rotate the straightened arms until you feel slight tension.
3. *Rotate the straightened arms in the other direction.* Rotate the straightened arms in the other direction until you feel slight tension and hold them there a few seconds.
4. *Rotate the arms back-and-forth, with the wrists bent back and fingers straightened.* With the wrist back and the fingers straightened, rotate the arms back-and-forth, feeling the sense of tension.
5. When you are tense, you can stretch both arms, or one arm, in this way. [The therapist should model the stretch with one arm.]
6. Repeat one or two more times if desired.

• Arm Relaxation: Bent-Arm Rotation Method

1. *Bend an arm.*
2. *Wrist rotation.* With the arm slightly bent, rotate at the wrist, doing this about two or three rotations.
3. *Finger wiggle.* Straighten and arch back the fingers, and then make back-and-forth wriggling motion with the fingers.
4. Repeat the wrist rotation and finger wiggle a few times.

• When to Practice Stretching

You should practice these stretches at the following times:

Practice upon Returning Home

When you go home today you should practice this, so you will not forget.

Practice before Bed

You should also practice each night before going to bed, for instance, while watching television.

Practice Stretching When You Are Upset

If you do it when you are upset, it will make you feel better. [Here could mention that *salah* may also be performed to feel better such as at the various times during the day in the time windows specified in the Islamic faith (e.g., before going to bed) or when feeling upset; could mention that the patient may remain in the various physical postures (e.g., bowing and prostrating) for an extended period (e.g., several seconds to minutes), which also stretches the body to make it more flexible and relaxed.]

Homework

• Stretching before Sleep

Practice the stretch we taught you today, in particular before going to bed. Use the handout to guide you while doing the stretches.

You can do the stretches while watching television before bed. (And you can do *salah* to improve bodily flexibility.)

• Muscle Tension Awareness and Applied Muscle Stretching

Muscle tension awareness. During the day, try to be aware of the tension in your body, and stretch any area of tightness. You should practice muscle stretching in some of the following situations:

○ *When tense.* If you feel tight in your body, in your mood.
○ *When in a bad mood state.* If you are in a bad mood.
○ *When in a difficult situation.* If you find it hard to adjust to a situation.

How to practice applied muscle stretching. If you notice tension in an area, stretch that area. For example, you can do the following:

○ Stretch the shoulders by rolling them.
○ Straighten and rotate arm.
○ Bend the arm and rotate at the wrist.
○ Wiggle the straightened fingers.
○ Rotate the wrist again.
○ Stretch any area of tension.
  [If the therapist notes an area of tightness in the patient, this should be stretched. The therapist can stretch any body area where he or she feels tightness; often this tightness comes from sensing tightness in the patient in that area.]

• A Box of Tools: To Be Used When Having Bad Memories or Feeling Anxious/Depressed upon Awakening from a Nightmare

Whenever you have bad memories, or when you are anxious or depressed or you have a nightmare, you can try any of the following. They are like a set of tools. You can use one of them, or all of them. Use what is helpful to you.

Try Different Emotions

Compassion. Try feeling compassion for yourself and others.

Bring Yourself into the Moment with All Your Senses

Attend to what is happening around you right now, in all your senses.

➢ Look at how leaves or branches move with each breeze.

Try to Stretch the Body

Stretch any place you feel tension, like in your jaw, opening the mouth, and moving the jaw from side to side. [The therapist should briefly enact this, rotating the head; opening the mouth and moving the jaw from side to side, thereby stretching the jaw; and straightening the arm, then rotating the arm this way and that.]

Do Something You Like

You may want to do something you like. You may want to take a walk or watch television

• Candle (and Incense) Imagery: Flexibility Primers[4]

Observing Candle Flames

This week, note how the flames of candles dance with each breeze and make ever-changing shapes, bending this way and that with each breeze or draft. [Could mention to note how incense or candle lights move, displaying flexibility, moving with each slight breeze; for example, they should observe incense in the Mosque if applicable.]

Paired Lesson

The deep lesson of the candle flame is to learn to adjust to each circumstance, to be flexible. The candle, its flame, is a symbol that reminds one to be flexible not rigid.

Noticing Candles and Possibly Purchasing a Votive Candle

Observe candles and their flames around you and remember that they are reminding you to be flexible.

You may want to buy a votive candle at a store. When you light it, watch how it dances in the breeze, and think of how the flame symbolizes flexibility.

• Multisensorial Living-in-the-Moment Homework

As you go home, we want you to practice the following, to practice living in the moment and attending to your senses (i.e., mindfulness), to what is around you right now, and practice this in the following week.

To Practice Upon Leaving the Office: Meditation Lesson

• Explanation for Performing Loving Kindness

We want you to practice having another feeling and to put your mind and focus on a good thing. We want you to practice having other types of emotion.

• Performing Loving Kindness

Water and cooling imagery[5]

❑ Upon leaving today, as you walk along, practice projecting sublime love to God, love to his prophets, and then love to all beings.[6]

---

[4] The therapist discusses candle flame (and incense) imagery in order to promote psychological and emotional flexibility.

[5] In Islamic tradition, water and cooling imagery is valued. The Quran narrates how the prophet Job (*Ayub,* in Arabic), who fell ill, was eventually instructed by God to strike his foot on the ground. This in turn caused cool and fresh healing waters to pour forth for him to drink and bathe in. In turn, Job became cured of all his sickness (Quran 38:41–43). Likewise, prophet Abraham was thrown into a fire, but miraculously survived as sudden coldness from God covered his body, "oh fire be you coolness and safety for Abraham" (Quran 21:69).

[6] This particular hierarchy of directing loving kindness is more in line with core Islamic values, with God being deserving of a form of ultimate love. Prophets are next in line as they belong to the spiritual realm and deserve a type of spiritual and transcendent love and admiration. Next, selfless love is directed to others, including family members, which is crucial according to Islam, a type of non-ego-based love. Such love should ideally first be directed towards parents, starting with the

- Loving kindness is a way to practice having a positive emotion.
- Direct love to Allah (or God) (a type of ultimate love); and thereafter his prophets (e.g., prophet Muhammad, and prophets such as Adam, Noh [i.e., Noah], Ibrahim [i.e., Abraham], Musa [i.e., Moses], and Eisa [i.e., Jesus]).
- Direct love and kindness to your parents (e.g., starting with your mother and then father) and then the rest of your family.[7]
- Direct love and kindness to the *ummah* (global Muslim community) and then all beings (global community in general).[8]
- Direct love and kindness to yourself.
- Imagine love flowing from your heart, like a cooling water.
- Imagine the water flowing out from your heart in all directions.
- Imagine that the water extinguishes all anger.
- Wish that all beings be happy.
- Wish that all beings be free from anger.
- Wish that all beings have wisdom.
- Imagine loving kindness flowing from your heart to all beings, like a water flowing from your heart.

Practice projecting a feeling of sublime love to God, and love and kindness to all beings as you go home, and during the next week. [Could mention here that one may supplicate for others (e.g., asking God to forgive them); e.g., mention that the Quran stresses the importance of supplicating for one's parents in particular, "My Lord, have mercy upon them [my parents] as they brought me up [when I was] small" (17:24), and that the Prophet encouraged the act of supplicating for others in general (a sign of mercy); e.g., he said "no Muslim supplicates for his brother behind his back but that the angel says: And for you the same,"[9] and "none of you has faith until he loves for his brother or neighbour what he loves for himself,"[10] and "Allah will not be merciful to those who are not merciful to mankind."[11] One could mention the importance of forgiving others if they have done you wrong; like prophet Muhammad (the role model for Muslims), who after he was physically abused said, "My Lord, forgive my people for they do not know"[12]; and as the Quran states that Muslims are those "who restrain [their] anger and who pardon the people and Allah loves the doers of good" (3:134). Finally, could mention here that the patient may make *tauba* for himself or herself (i.e., asking God for forgiveness).]

---

mother and then the father (and then remaining family members); then the *ummah* (*Muslim community*), and then mankind.

[7] The Quran stresses the importance of showing parents mercy, especially the mother; for instance, "lower to them [i.e., your parents] the wing of humility out of mercy and say, 'My Lord, have mercy upon them as they brought me up [when I was] small'", and "We [i.e., God] have enjoined upon man [to take good care] for his parents His mother carried him, [increasing her] in weakness upon weakness, and his weaning is in two years. Be grateful to Me [i.e., God] and to your parents." These Quranic verses and sayings of the Prophet may be mentioned to patients.

[8] This order of showing love and kindness is consistent with the Prophet's teachings that Muslims globally belong to a special brotherhood/sisterhood (*ummah*); e.g., "the Muslims are like a single man. If the eye is afflicted, then the whole body is afflicted. If the head is afflicted, then the whole body is afflicted."

[9] Found in the Muslim collection.   [10] See Sahih al-Bukhari.   [11] See Sahih al-Bukhari.

[12] Found in the Muslim collection.

Session

4

Education about Anxious-Depressive Distress, Modifying Catastrophic Cognitions, and Teaching Emotional Distancing

Overview of Core Lessons

In this session, metaphors are presented to educate about anxious-depressive distress and to help emotional processing: the "inner child watching DVDs" analogy and "two-television sets" analogy. Catastrophic cognitions about symptoms of distress are addressed: the patient is taught about the physiology of fear. Emotional processing is practiced.

Outline of Session 4
- Homework review
- Emotion Regulation Practice
  - Practicing the Dysphoria (Anxiety/Depression) Protocol
  - Practicing the Bad Memory Protocol (Emotion Regulation Toolbox)
- Core Lessons
  1. Education about bad memories and how to handle it using analogy of the inner child watching DVDs
  2. Modify catastrophic cognitions about distress symptoms
  3. Practice an emotion regulation technique: emotional distancing
- Stretching module for before bed
  - Behind-the-back, straight-arm stretch
  - Above-the-head, straight-arm stretch
  - Shoulder roll stretch
  - Standing, straight-leg-type stretch
- Homework
  - Stretching before sleep
  - Muscle-tension awareness and applied stretching
  - Mood distancing
  - Exercise
  - Practice smiling mindfulness
  - Week's meditation lesson

52

- Meditation upon returning home
  - ○ Leaf movement, shape, and color mindfulness
  - ○ Cloud movement, shape, and color mindfulness
  - ○ Mindful eating

Homework Review

Living in the Moment upon Returning Home

As you went home at the end of the last session, and during the last week, did you practice living in the moment, paying attention to how leaves and branches moved in the wind?

Stretching before Sleep

Last week did you practice stretching each night before going to sleep? Do you have the sheet showing the stretches, or do you need a new one?

Explore Recent Distress Episodes

Distress in the last week. Did you feel anxious, depressed, or upset at any time this last week? If so, when and why?

Self-treatment of distress. Did you do anything that helped you when you were anxious or depressed?

Practicing the Dysphoria (Anxiety/Depression) Protocol

If you are anxious, depressed, or upset, you can do any of the following to feel better:

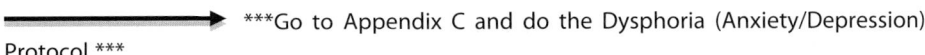 ***Go to Appendix C and do the Dysphoria (Anxiety/Depression) Protocol ***

Bad Memory Check

• Explore Recent Bad Memories

Presence of Bad Memories

In the last week, did you have any recall of the past when you didn't want to, either when awake or during a nightmare? If so, please describe.[1] [If the patient had no bad memories in the last week, then ask about the most recent episode.]

Presence of Flashback

Was your recall vivid, as if it were happening again? If so, please describe.

---

[1] Through this, and the following questions, the goal is to have the patient, or a member of the group, share some bad memories. If a patient admits to bad memories, and becomes visibly upset, the patient should be told not to recount the event at this moment, and one should begin the "Bad Memory Protocol" (Appendix D).

• Elicitation of Self-Treatment of Bad Memory

When you had the bad memory, did you do anything to feel better?

Practicing the Bad Memory Protocol (Tools to Use upon Having Bad Memories or When Distressed)

When you have bad memories, or feel distressed, you can do any of the following. These are some tools you can use. Use whichever part you want to use.

⟶ ***Go to Appendix D and do the Bad Memory Protocol (Emotion Regulation Toolbox)***

Core Lesson 1: Education about Anxious-Depressive Distress and How to Manage Bad Memories Using the Inner Child Watching DVD Analogy

It is normal and common to encounter something that reminds you of the past. Sometimes you may not even know that you feel angry or sad or scared because something has reminded you of a bad thing that happened in the past.

• Triggering of Bad Memories Compared to an Inner Child Watching a DVD of the Past

Inner Child Recalls All

It is as if you have an inner child that remembers all the bad things that happened to you in the past.

Inner Child Has DVDs of Distressing Events

It is as if the child has a TV with a DVD player. Next to the DVD player are hundreds of DVDs, each of which represents a bad event in the past. In a tall cabinet are DVD recordings of all the scary and frightening things you have ever experienced.

Inner Child Plays the DVDs When Anything Recalls the Past

If anything occurs now that is like one of those past bad events, the "inner child" may play that "bad event" DVD. That is, if anything happens around you, the inner child will yell out, "Hey, this is just like when this or that bad thing happened. It will happen again."

Then the inner child will insert the DVD of the disturbing event. Soon your heart begins to pound and you become frightened.

What Reminds the Inner Child of the Past: Taking-Out-Similar-DVDs Examples

The following may remind the inner child of a bad thing from the past; may cause the inner child to take out and play a video of an earlier bad event:

Rain example. In the present moment, it may be raining. This may cause the inner child to take out a DVD of a bad thing that happened on a rainy day.

Dizziness example. If you get a little dizzy, or feel some other uncomfortable physical sensation in your body, it may cause the inner child to pull out a DVD of when you were dizzy and a bad thing happened, as when you were hit in the head.

Fear example. If you are afraid, the inner child will pull out DVDs of times when you were afraid in the past, of bad things that caused you to feel afraid in the past.

• What to Do When Having Bad Memories: Framed in Terms of the Inner Child Watching DVDs of the Past

Comfort the Scared Inner Child: Come into the Present Moment

If you remember a bad thing from the past, tell the inner child something like the following: "This is now, that was then. Stop watching DVDs of the past, stop viewing those old DVDs. Live in the present moment, enjoy the present moment."

Comfort the Scared Inner Child: Be Gentle with It

- ○ Comfort the inner child, be gentle with yourself.
- ○ Sing to the inner child, comfort it.

Comfort the Scared Inner Child: Tell the Child to Play Good-Memory DVDs

Tell the inner child that if he or she must watch old DVDs, then put in DVDs about the good things that happened in the past. Tell the inner, scared child to watch joyful DVDs.

Rain example (good DVD). If it rains outside, have the inner child play a DVD of good things that happened on a rainy day, like playing in the rain as a child.

Dizziness example (good DVD). If you get dizzy, have the inner child think of times you felt so happy when you were dizzy, like when you rolled down a hill as a child, the joy and dizziness you felt.

Further Inner-Child Metaphors to Promote a Sense of Shift: Television Example

Changing channels. Tell the inner child to change the channel, to switch the channel from the bad event to a happier image on another channel.

Watching several channels. At the very least, have the inner child watch the good and bad channels at the same time, flipping between them.

Watching several televisions. Or imagine two televisions, one playing the upsetting event, the other playing an event you like. Have the inner child watch both televisions, or even many televisions.

Contemplating paradise channel. The Quran utilizes vivid imagery of paradise (in Arabic *jannah*) as a way to shift attentional and emotional focus onto a positive object. As an example, "Those will have gardens of perpetual residence; beneath them rivers will flow. They will be adorned therein with bracelets of gold and will wear green garments of fine silk and brocade, reclining therein on adorned couches. Excellent is the reward, and good is the resting place" (18:31); and "Those will have a provision determined – fruits; and they will be honored. In gardens of pleasure. On thrones facing one another. There will be circulated among them a cup [of wine] from a flowing spring. White and delicious to the drinkers" (37:41–46). Or too the

Prophet said, "[In paradise are] bricks of gold and silver, mortar of fragrant musk, pebbles of pearl and sapphire, and soil of saffron. Whoever enters it is filled with joy and will never feel miserable; he will live there forever and will never die; their clothes will never wear out and their youth will never fade."[2] The Quran stipulates that such pleasures are rewarded to those who are patient and steadfast, for example, persevere during times of hardship: "And no soul knows what has been hidden for them of comfort for eyes as reward [i.e., paradise] for what they used to do" (32:17). [Such Quranic and prophetic descriptions of paradise can be mentioned to patients as a way to shift attentional focus and promote positive affect and expectation for the future (i.e., to tackle hopelessness and despair).]

Core Lesson 2: Modifying Catastrophic Cognitions about Distress Symptoms

• Modifying Catastrophic Cognitions about Physical-Type Anxiety Symptoms

Somatic Symptoms Triggered by a Bad Memory or Anxiety or Depression

When you are reminded of the past, or get anxious, depressed, or upset, it is normal if you get symptoms like:

- ➢ palpitations
- ➢ shortness of breath
- ➢ sweating
- ➢ dizziness
- ➢ ringing in the ears
- ➢ upset in the stomach
- ➢ shaking of the arms and legs

Modifying Catastrophic Cognitions about Physical-Type Symptoms of Anxiety or Depression

There is no danger. Do not worry. These symptoms will not kill you, will not harm you. They are just from anxiety or depression. Once you learn to relax, these symptoms will improve.

Elicit Autonomic Arousal Symptoms, the Embodiment of Distress

When you are afraid, what symptoms do you get that bother you?

Elicit Catastrophic Cognitions

Do these sensations make you afraid there is something wrong with your body or mind? If so, what are you afraid of, and why?

---

[2] Narration found in the at-Tirmidhi collection.

Address Those Catastrophic Cognitions

These symptoms result from fear, and are not dangerous. [The therapist should provide education about the symptoms, modifying catastrophic cognitions.]

• Modifying Catastrophic Cognitions about Mental-Type Anxiety or Depression Symptoms

Mental Symptoms Triggered by Bad Memories, Anxiety or Depression

When you are reminded of the past, or you are anxious, depressed, or upset, it is normal if you get symptoms like:

➢ racing thoughts
➢ being unable to concentrate
➢ being forgetful

Modifying Catastrophic Cognitions about Mental-Type Anxiety or Depression Symptoms

There is no danger. Do not worry. These symptoms will not kill you. They are just from distress. Once you learn to relax, these symptoms will improve.

Elicit Autonomic Arousal Symptoms, the Embodiment of Distress

When you are afraid, what symptoms do you get that bother you, like symptoms in your body?

Elicit Catastrophic Cognitions

Do these symptoms make you afraid there is something wrong with your body or mind? If so, what are you afraid of, and why?

Address Those Catastrophic Cognitions

Symptoms like these are from anxiety or depression and are not dangerous. [The therapist should provide education about the symptom, modifying catastrophic cognitions.]

• Review the Salient Cultural Syndromes and Modify Related Catastrophic Cognitions

When you get anxiety or depression symptoms, such as shortness of breath or dizziness or palpitations, you may fear something is wrong with you, that you have a disorder. But there is no danger.

Core Lesson 3: Practicing an Emotion Regulation Technique: Emotional Distancing

• An Observational, Detached Viewing

If you have an emotion or thought, especially an unpleasant one, just observe the emotion or thought. Just let it be. Watch it. Maintain distance from your mood and thoughts, watching them. Studying them.

• An Observational Metaphor: Emotions in the Mind Are Like Clouds in the Sky

Emotions will pass away like clouds from the sky. Emotions are like clouds floating in the sky. Simply let them pass, just as clouds pass across the sky. Our minds are like the sky while our emotions resemble the clouds. Soon the emotion will pass away.

Study the emotion as you would study clouds. Examine the emotion much as you would examine the color of a cloud, or the cloud's shape, or the cloud's movement.

Soon another emotion will come. Soon the cloud will pass out of the sky; soon the emotion will pass out of your mind. Soon another mood will arrive. Simply watch your emotions, staying apart from them, watching them like clouds in the sky.

• Practice Labeling Emotions and Detached and Curious Observation

❑ *Notice your emotion.* Be aware of your emotions.

❑ *Label your emotion.* Observe your mood, and label it, whether the emotion is anger, fear, worry, envy, disgust, anxiety, happiness, or excitement.

❑ *Cloud analogy.* Watch your thoughts and moods like you would observe clouds passing across the sky.

❑ *Detached and curious observation.* Just watch your mood, not acting on it, looking at it like it's a cloud in the sky, which will soon pass away. Observe your moods in a detached and curious way, distance yourself from your emotion, observing it.

Week's Stretching Module with a Paired Instructional Metaphor

• Introduction to Stretching

We want to teach you how to stretch. Each week we will teach you to stretch.

• Handout of Stretching

All the stretches are in a handout with pictures to remind you how to do the stretching. Do you still have that handout? [If not, give to the patient.]

• Rationale for Stretching

Help Sleep

It will help you to sleep because it
○ will help you relax
○ will prevent cramps

Flexible Body, Flexible Mind

If you are more relaxed and flexible in your body, it will help you to be more relaxed and more flexible in your emotions, mind, and ways of thinking.

Help make you feel better when upset

If you stretch when upset, it will make you feel better.

• Embodying Metaphors

While doing the stretching, think the following [the therapist can repeat this while the stretching is being done]:

➤ "As I become more flexible in my body, may I become more flexible in my thoughts, in my emotions, may I know how to adjust to each new situation." [Or, "Oh Allah may I become more flexible in my body, may I become more flexible in my thoughts, in my emotions, may I know how to adjust to each new situation."]

• Relaxing the Shoulders: Behind-the-Back, Straight-Arm Stretch

1. Stand.
2. Put the arms behind your back.
3. Grasp the hands together, the fingers interlocking.
4. Straighten the arms.
5. Keeping the arms straight, and the hands clasped, raise the arms until you feel a little tension.
6. Hold the arms there and count to ten slowly.
7. Unclasp the hands, and let the arms fall to your side.
8. Repeat one or two more times if desired.

• Relaxing the Shoulders: Above-the-Head, Straight-Arm Stretch

1. Stand.
2. Put your two arms forward and straight ahead and then grasp the hands together, the fingers interlocking.
3. Straighten the arms, producing a little tension, all the while keeping the hands clasped together.
4. Keeping the arms straight and the hands clasped together, make an upward arc by raising them upwards above the head.
5. Reach up as far as you can so that you straighten your body and spine and arms, creating a pulling feeling.
6. Keeping the arms straight and the hands clasped together, bend from one side to another, slowly, feeling the pulling tension in the arms.
7. Do this two or three times, one side and then another, all the while making sure to pull up, to reach as high as possible.
8. Unclasp the hands, and let the arms fall to your side.
9. Repeat one or two more times if desired.

• Relaxing the Shoulders: Rolling-the-Shoulders Stretch

1. Stand.
2. Roll the shoulders forward.
3. Roll the shoulders back.
4. Roll the shoulders forward.
5. Roll the shoulders back.
6. Try to tighten the stomach muscles a little as you do it.
7. Repeat one or two more times if desired.

• Stretching the Legs: Standing, Straight-Leg Type

1. Stand facing a wall (or a door) that has nothing on it.
2. Put both hands on the wall.
3. With the arms so positioned, the legs should be slightly apart, parallel to one another, and pointing straight to the wall. [The feet should be at a 90 degree angle to the wall.]
4. Put one leg out behind the other.
5. With that leg straight, bend the other leg.
6. Stop the bending when stretching is felt in the straight leg.
7. Hold the stretching position while counting to ten slowly.
8. Now switch legs, repeating the above.
9. Both legs should be stretched as described, up to three times.

• When to Practice Stretching

You should practice these stretches at the following times:

Practice Stretching upon Returning Home

When you get home, practice the stretching we taught you today. Do each stretch three times.

Practice Stretching Every Night Before Bed

Every night, before you go to bed, for example when you are watching television, practice the stretches we have taught you.

Practice Stretching When You Are Upset

If you do it when you are upset, it will make you feel better. [Here could mention that *salah* may also be performed to feel better such as at the various times during the day in the time windows specified in the Islamic faith (e.g., before going to bed) or when feeling upset; could mention that the patient may remain in the various physical postures (e.g., bowing and prostrating) for an extended period (e.g., several seconds to minutes), which also stretches the body to make it more flexible and relaxed.]

Homework

• Stretching before Sleep

Practice the stretch we taught you today, in particular before going to bed. Use the handout to guide you when doing the stretches.

You can do the stretches while watching television before bed. [And you can do *salah* to improve bodily flexibility]

• Muscle Tension Awareness and Applied Muscle Stretching

During the day, try to be aware of the tension in your body, and then stretch any area of tightness. For example, you can stretch the shoulders:

➢ Relax the shoulders
  ○ Stretch the shoulders by rolling them.
  ○ Roll the head on the shoulders.

[If the therapist notes an area of tightness in the patient, this should be stretched. The therapist can stretch any body area where he or she feels tight, because this tightness comes from sensing tightness in the patient.]

• Practice in Mood Distancing: Cloud analogy

Try to observe your emotions and thoughts as if they are clouds in the sky. Soon they will pass out of the mind, like a cloud across the sky. Try to observe them; stay at a distance from them.

• Exercise

Try to exercise this week. It will help you get better. You may want to take a walk, or do some other exercises.

• Practice Smiling (Facial-Expression Mindfulness)

Practice Having a Slight Smile

This week, try to practice having a slight smile whenever you meet and talk to someone. For example, have a slight smile on your face as you pass by or interact with strangers (e.g., at the grocery store or train station). Also, have a slight smile on your face when you interact with your family at home. [Here the therapist should remind the patient that the prophet Muhammad, who is the role model for all Muslims to emulate as per the Quran, where it is written that "surely there was a good example for you in the Messenger of Allah," i.e., prophet Muhammad (33:21), who was seen smiling often, and notably said that "smiling in the face of your brother is charity."]

Explanation for Why You Should Do This

Improve your own mood. This will improve your own mood.
Others will not think you are mad at them or don't like them. If you don't smile, you may frown, and others will think you are mad at them or that you don't like them.

Notice the Interpersonal Effects

If you smile this week, notice whether people react to you in a different way.

• Meditation Homework

As you go home, we want you to practice the following lesson, putting your mind on good things, and we'd like you to practice this all week. It is also a way to practice living in the moment with all your senses.

To Practice Upon Leaving the Office: Meditation Lesson

• How the Attentional Object Determines Mood[3]

What you put your mind on will determine your mood, how you feel. Put your mind on a good object, on something that will improve your mood. For example, the Muslim religion teaches many ways to put the mind on God to enter a better state. [Here the therapist can

---

[3] Remember to maintain a relaxed mood when teaching meditation, slowing down and deepening the voice to create a sense of relaxation.

mention: (1) *dhikr* (i.e., engaging in the remembrance of Allah), e.g., through pondering Allah's names such as The Ever Forgiving and The Most Loving; (2) *dua* (i.e., supplicating); (3) *tasbeeh* (repeating each of three distinct praises of God thirty-three or thirty-four times as appropriate while using the fingers to count); (4) *salah* (ritualistic prayer), done with complete attentional focus on God (i.e., *kushoo*); (5) reciting the Quran; (6) doing *ruqyah* (e.g., by reciting Quranic verses and then gently blowing on various parts of his/her own body); and (7) doing *wudhu* (ritualistic washing) while mindful of water running down the limbs and cleansing off sins.]

• Explanation for Practicing Present-Moment Awareness (Mindfulness)

Keep your mind on good objects. Pay attention to what is going on around you as you head home. Noticing all the sounds, colors, and movements in the moment, will keep your mind on good things.

Prevent your mind from floating to the past, floating to the future. By paying attention to something going on around you right now, your mind will not float to the past, to the future, to upsetting thoughts and concerns.

Don't miss the beauty around you. Often we walk along, we think of this problem or that or feel angry towards something or someone, and we forget to look at the beauty of what is around us. We are thinking about this or that, feeling angry about something, are in our heads, and we walk by something beautiful, say a beautiful tree or a beautiful colored leaf, and don't even notice it. We are in our heads, in our thoughts, in our anger, and fail to notice what is going on around us. [A way to promote such sensorial awareness is by asking patients to contemplate the beauty of God's creation such as clouds, trees, and how the leaves move with the wind.]

• Leaf Mindfulness

When you go home today, practice living in the moment with all the senses in the following way, and practice this in the following week. Note what is going on around you. [Point outside if there are trees or clouds visible]:

Visual Modality: Leaves

Leaf movement. Note how the leaves, and branches, move in the wind.

Leaf shape. Note the shape of the leaves (or branches if there are no leaves).

Leaf color. Note the color of the leaves (or branches and tree trunk if there are no leaves).

Light and shadow on leaf. Note the light and shadow on leaves.

• Cloud Mindfulness

Visual Modality: Clouds

Cloud movement. Note how the clouds move across the sky.

Cloud shape. Note the shape of the clouds.

Cloud color. Note the color of the clouds, the whiteness or grey, the color of the sky.

• Mindful Eating

When you are home today pay special attention to the foods you eat. Pay full attention to their rich flavors, smells, and textures with all your senses. [Here the therapist can mention that the prophet Muhammad said, "when one of you eats some food, let him say *Bismillah* (i.e., in the name of God)," and also taught his followers to praise Allah upon finishing eating; for instance, "Allah is pleased with His servant when he eats something and praises Him for it, or drinks something and praises Him for it." Can also mention that the Prophet stressed the importance of not overeating; for instance, he said, "a man does not fill any vessel worse than his stomach." The therapist may remind the patient of the overall benefits of not overeating (e.g., energy, weight loss, and reduced bodily inflammation). The therapist can mention occasional fasting (e.g., one to two times a week) as an option (i.e., if the patient is otherwise healthy and accustomed to fasting during *ramadhan*); mention that the Prophet, in addition to the month of *ramadhan,* used to fast every Monday and Thursday, and that such fasting makes the body lighter and reduces laziness. It also makes one more grateful for food (i.e., upon breaking the fast). Mention that the patient should pay special attention to (i.e., fully concentrate on) the fast-breaking foods with all the senses (e.g., their flavors, smells, and textures).]

Interoceptive Exposure I: Head Rotation

Overview of Core Lessons

Interoceptive exposure is introduced, focusing on dizziness sensations that are induced by head rolling. There is also the creation of positive associations to dizziness sensations and addressing of catastrophic cognitions about them. We use head rolling to educate about dizziness, to create positive reassociations to dizziness and other induced sensations, to address distress associations to the induced symptoms, to reduce fears of dizziness and other induced symptoms, and to act as interoceptive exposure that creates new nonthreatening associations to the induced symptoms. Interoceptive exposure also acts as behavioral activation as well as promoting an attitude of playfulness, a sort of flexibility. There is also further training in emotion regulation (emotion flexibility) by practicing certain emotions.

Outline of Session 5

- Homework review
- Distress check (review of the Dysphoria [Anxiety/Depression] Protocol)
- Bad memory check (review of the Bad Memory Protocol [Emotion Regulation Toolbox])
- Core lesson
  1. Head rolling
     - ➤ Introducing head rolling
     - ➤ Positive associations to dizziness
     - ➤ Performing head rolling

  2. Practicing emotions
     - ➤ Compassion
     - ➤ Joy in the joy of others
     - ➤ Loving kindness
     - ➤ Detached, curious observer

- Stretching module before bed
  - ○ Behind-the-back, straight-arm stretch
  - ○ Above-the-head, straight-arm stretch
  - ○ Rolling shoulders
  - ○ Standing, straight-leg stretch
  - ○ Standing, bent-leg stretch

- Homework:
  - Stretching before sleep
  - Muscle tension awareness and applied stretching
  - Head rolling and reassociation
  - Practicing belly laughing
  - Week's meditation module
- Meditation upon returning home and during the coming week
  - Leaf movement paired with an instructional metaphor
  - Mindful eating

Homework Review

Living in the Moment upon Returning Home

As you went home at the end of the last session, and during the last week, did you practice living in the moment, paying attention to how leaves and branches moved in the wind?

Stretching before Sleep

Last week did you practice stretching each night before going to sleep? Do you have the sheet showing the stretches, or do you need a new one?

Explore Recent Distress Episodes

Distress in the last week. Did you feel anxious, depressed, or upset at any time this last week? If so, when and why?

Self-treatment of distress. Did you do anything that helped you when you were anxious/depressed?

Practicing the Dysphoria (Anxiety/Depression) Protocol

If you are anxious, depressed, or upset, you can do any of the following to feel better:

⟶ ***Go to Appendix C and do the Dysphoria (Anxiety/Depression) Protocol***

Bad Memory Check

- ## Explore Recent Bad Memories

Presence of Bad Memories

In the last week, did you have any recall of the past when you didn't want to, either when awake or during a nightmare? If so, please describe.[1] [If the patient had no bad memories in the last week, then ask about the most recent episode.]

---

[1] As described above, have the patient describe the bad memories to the point of being slightly upset. If the patient is very upset, immediately start the "Bad Memory Protocol" (Appendix D).

Presence of Flashback

Was your recall vivid, as if it were happening again? If so, please describe.

• Elicitation of Self-Treatment of Bad Memories

When you had the bad memories, did you do anything to feel better?

Practicing the Bad Memory Protocol (Tools to Use upon Having Bad Memories or When Distressed)

When you have bad memories, or feel distressed, you can do any of the following. These are some tools you can use. Use whichever part you want to use:

⟶ ***Go to Appendix D and do the Bad Memory Protocol (Emotion Regulation Toolbox)***

Core Lesson 1: Head Rolling

• Introducing Head Rolling

Head Rolling as a Game

We now will have you spin your head and practice thinking of good things when you are dizzy. It is a game. We want to do this so you learn not to be afraid of dizziness and other feelings you have in your body.

Have Good Images Come to Mind When You Are Dizzy

We want you to think of good things when you have dizziness and when you have other sensations in your body.

• Modifying Catastrophic Cognitions about Head Spinning

We want to explain the following, so that when you spin your head, you will not be afraid:[2]

- *Even if you have high blood pressure, it is safe to rotate the head.* If your neck is sore, if your blood pressure is high, turning your head is still completely safe.
- *Sounds heard upon rotating the head are from tendons and muscles: there is no danger.* If you hear a sound when you turn your head, do not worry; there is no danger. The sound is made by muscles and tendons. You are stretching your muscles and it makes that sound.
- *Rotating the head is completely safe.* If you turn your head rapidly, if you spin it, it is completely safe.
- *Normal to get dizziness.* If you get dizziness, or get other symptoms, as you roll the head, it does not indicate any problem.

---

[2] In very rare cases, the patient could have some problem with the spine or neck that prevents doing this exercise, such as an old injury. Be sure to inquire about this prior to beginning lesson.

• Promoting Positive (and Adaptive) Associations to Head Spinning

Game Analogy: Head Spinning Game

Play with the dizziness, make it a game, "the head-spinning game."

Analogy to DVD-Watching Child: Good Dizziness Videos

As you get dizzy, have the inner child put in good DVDs about dizziness. As you turn your head and feel a little dizzy, think of the following:

- *Rolling down a hill:* of rolling down a hill like a child playing a game.
- *Riding a roller coaster:* of a roller coaster – it is something that people pay money to ride because they like to become dizzy or queasy.
- *Standing-and-spinning game:* of how children like to spin in circles, just to experience being dizzy.
- *Being happy until dizzy:* of when you felt so happy you were dizzy.
- *Running and playing until dizzy:* of playing and running until you were dizzy.
- *Playing traditional games:* of playing other games as a child that made you dizzy, such as . . .

[Here you can mention culturally appropriate activities and games. Ask patients to recall when they were children and played such games; how they felt dizzy and also happy]

- *Being flexible:* of dizziness being a reminder to do the following:
  - ➤ To turn and consider all the possible roads, to be flexible, to consider all the possibilities. [The therapist should turn the head from side to side when saying this.]

• Performing Head Rolling

Framing Head Rolling as a Game

We are now going to play the head rotation game. Play and enjoy the game of rolling your head, the "rolling the head" game!

Doing Head Rolling

Initial instructions. Roll the head like I am doing now. Faster and faster until you are dizzy. Enjoy it. It is a game. There is no danger. Enjoy it!

[The therapist rolls the head. The therapist should observe how quickly the patient rotates the head, whether there is hesitation and fear. If there is hesitation, encourage the patient to rotate the head more quickly, framing the head rolling as a game, assuring the patient it is completely safe, mentioning some positive associations to dizziness, such as "rolling down a hill."]

Articulating joy during head rolling. See, it is fun, "weee." [Have the patient do head rolling for about 30–60 seconds. When doing the head rolling, the therapist should act as if it is very enjoyable, even making a sound like "weee . . ."]

• Asking about Induced Symptoms, Catastrophic Cognitions, and Distress Associations

Did Spinning Your Head Make You Afraid?

Did head spinning make you afraid? If so, why? [If the patient does endorse fear, address those concerns.]

Eliciting Head-Rotation-Induced Somatic Symptoms

What symptoms did you have while spinning your head?

Address Catastrophic Cognitions about Induced Somatic Symptoms

Did those sensations make you afraid?

Query about Dizziness

Did you feel dizzy? Were you afraid? Why? [If so, address catastrophic cognitions.]

Query about Bad Memories

When you were rolling your head, did any memories of the past come into your mind? If so, which memories? [If the patient has severe bad memories, consider doing the Bad Memory Protocol.]

• Positive Reassociation to Dizziness

Tell the Inner Child That It's Not Dangerous

Try to teach the inner child that dizziness is not dangerous, that these sensations are not dangerous. Have fun with them! Play with them!

Good Associations to Dizziness

Remember when as a child you liked to make yourself dizzy. Remember good things associated with making yourself dizzy. Put in a good DVD of dizziness such as:

❖ Rolling down a hill as a child.
❖ Running until you were short of breath and dizzy, falling to the ground and laughing, laying on your back and looking up at the clouds in the sky.

• **Repeat Head Rotation One More Time**

Framing Head Rolling as a Game

We are now going to play the head rotation game again. Play and enjoy the game of rolling your head, the "rolling the head" game!

Doing Head Rolling

Initial Instructions. Roll the head like I am doing now. Faster and faster until you are dizzy. Enjoy it. It is a game. There is no danger. Enjoy it.

[The therapist should observe how quickly the patient rotates the head, whether there is hesitation and fear. If there is hesitation, encourage the patient to rotate the head more quickly, framing the head rolling as a game, assuring the patient it is completely safe, mentioning some positive associations to dizziness, such as "rolling down a hill."]

Articulating joy during head rolling. See, it is fun, "weee." [Have the patient do head rolling for about 30–60 seconds. When doing the head rolling, the therapist should act as if it is very enjoyable, even making sound like "weee . . . "]

• Education about Dizziness and Promoting Positive Associations

How Dizziness Occurs

Dizziness may be caused by many things:
- ❖ turning the head
- ❖ looking at many things that are moving
- ❖ distress or fear

Modifying Catastrophic Cognitions

This dizziness is not dangerous. It is not caused by a health problem.

Positive Reassociations

When you get a little dizzy, think of good things and have the inner child play memories of good things that involve dizziness:

- ❑ *Games.* Childhood memories of playing games as a child to induce dizziness
  - . like standing and spinning in place
  - . like running and playing as a child
  - . like rolling down a hill as a child

- ❑ *Turning your head to see all the roads.* Let the dizziness remind you to turn and look at all the roads, to look at all the possibilities.

Core Lesson 2: Practicing Emotions

Rationale for Practicing Various Emotions

Stuck on Certain Emotions

Sometimes we forget to practice having different emotions. We get stuck with one emotion, like anger, envy, regret, or worry.

Lack of Emotional Range: Comparison to Cooking, Painting, and Music

You want to practice having different emotions. Otherwise, you are like:
- ❖ A painter using only one or two colors.

❖ A cook using just one or two ingredients.
❖ A musician playing the same two notes.

• Practicing Emotion Shifting: Try Practicing these Following Emotions

Here are six emotions that research has shown will help you to be happy, that you should practice. Try one. [After giving each example, the therapist should pause; the therapist should speak slowly; this gives the patient time to imagine having the emotion]:

➢ *Compassion.* A feeling of compassion for the suffering of all beings.
➢ *Joy in the joy of others.* A feeling of joy when others are successful or happy.
➢ *Loving kindness.* A feeling of loving kindness toward yourself and all beings.
➢ *Gratitude.* A feeling of gratitude for the beauty of nature, for those who have helped you, for the things you have.
➢ *Forgiveness.* Forgive those who have caused you any pain. [May mention here that the Quran strongly encourages forgiving others; e.g., "so forgive with gracious forgiveness" (15:85), and the Prophet said, "forgive others and Allah will forgive you."[3]]
➢ *Detached, curious observation.*
   ○ *Observation and non-action.* A feeling of observing and letting go of all emotions, of just watching your emotions, of not acting on them, a feeling of non-judging, of waiting and watching your emotions. Stay distant from your emotions and strive for a state of curious observation.
   ○ *Label and observe effects.* Just label the emotion, look at the effects of the emotion on your thoughts and body, and let it go, stay distant from it. Say to yourself, "Oh, I have anger, and I will watch it, will stay distant from it, will let it go, rather than acting on it."
   ○ *Comparison of a mood to a cloud.* Like clouds in the sky, so too new thoughts and emotions will come to you. Just watch them, stay at a distance, and soon they will pass, like clouds from the sky.

Week's Stretching Module with a Paired Instructional Metaphor

• Introduction to Stretching

We want to teach you how to stretch. Each week we will teach you to stretch.

• Handout of Stretching

All the stretches are in a handout with pictures to remind you how to do the stretching. Do you still have that handout? [If not, give to the patient.]

• Rationale for Stretching

Help Sleep

It will help you to sleep because it

---

[3] Narration found in Musnad Ahmad.

- ○ will help you relax
- ○ will prevent cramps

Flexible Body, Flexible Mind
If you are more relaxed and flexible in your body, it will help you to be more relaxed and more flexible in your emotions, mind, and ways of thinking.

Help Make You Feel Better when Upset
If you stretch when upset, it will make you feel better.

• Embodying Metaphors
While doing the stretching, think the following [the therapist can repeat this while the stretching is being done]:

> "As I become more flexible in my body, may I become more flexible in my thoughts, in my emotions, may I know how to adjust to each new situation." [Or, "Oh Allah may I become more flexible in my body, may I become more flexible in my thoughts, in my emotions, may I know how to adjust to each new situation."]

• Relaxing the Shoulders: Behind-the-back, Straight-Arm Stretch
1. Stand.
2. Put the arms behind your back.
3. Grasp the hands together, the fingers interlocking.
4. Straighten the arms.
5. Keeping the arms straight, and the hands clasped, raise the arms until you feel a little tension.
6. Hold the arms there and count to ten slowly.
7. Unclasp the hands, and let the arms fall to your side.
8. Repeat one or two more times if desired.

• Relaxing the Shoulders: Above-the-Head, Straight-Arm Stretch
1. Stand.
2. Put your two arms forward and straight ahead and then grasp the hands together, the fingers interlocking.
3. Straighten the arms, producing a little tension, all the while keeping the hands clasped together.
4. Keeping the arms straight and the hands clasped together, make an upward arc by raising them upwards above the head.
5. Reach up as far as you can so that you straighten your body and spine and arms, creating a pulling feeling.
6. Keeping the arms straight and the hands clasped together, bend from one side to another, slowly, feeling the pulling tension in the arms.
7. Do this two or three times, one side and then another, all the while making sure to pull up, to reach as high as possible.
8. Unclasp the hands, and let the arms fall to your side.
9. Repeat one or two more times if desired.

• Relaxing the Shoulders: Rolling-the-Shoulders Stretch

1. Stand.
2. Roll the shoulders forward.
3. Roll the shoulders back.
4. Roll the shoulders forward.
5. Roll the shoulders back.
6. Try to tighten the stomach muscles a little as you do it.
7. Repeat one or two more times if desired.

• Stretching the Legs: Standing, Straight-Leg Type

1. Stand facing a wall (or a door) that has nothing on it.
2. Put both hands on the wall.
3. With the arms so positioned, the legs should be slightly apart, parallel to one another, and pointing straight to the wall. [The feet should be at a 90 degree angle to the wall.]
4. Put one leg out behind the other.
5. With that leg straight, bend the other leg.
6. Stop the bending when stretching is felt in the straight leg.
7. Hold the stretching position while counting to ten slowly.
8. Now switch legs, repeating the above.
9. Both legs should be stretched as described, up to three times.

• Stretching the Legs: Standing, Bent-Leg Type

1. Stand facing a wall (or a door) that has nothing on it.
2. Put both hands on the wall.
3. With the arms so positioned, the legs should be slightly apart, parallel to one another, and pointing straight to the wall. [The feet should be at a 90 degree angle to the wall.]
4. Put one leg out behind the other.
5. Bend down both legs, slowly.
6. Stop the bending when stretching is felt in the calf.
7. Hold the stretching position while counting to ten slowly.
8. Now switch legs, repeating the above.
9. Both legs should be stretched this time, up to three times [for this session, repeat one more time, for a total of two times].

• When to Practice Stretching

You should practice these stretches at the following times:

Practice Stretching upon Returning Home

When you get home, practice the stretching we taught you today. Do each stretch three times.

Practice Stretching Every Night before Bed

Every night, before you go to bed, for example when you are watching television, practice the stretches we have taught you.

Practice Stretching When You Are Upset

If you do it when you are upset, it will make you feel better. [Here could mention that *salah* may also be performed to feel better such as at the various times during the day in the time windows specified in the Islamic faith (e.g., before going to bed) or when feeling upset; could mention that the patient may remain in the various physical postures (e.g., bowing and prostrating) for an extended period (e.g., several seconds to minutes), which also stretches the body to make it more flexible and relaxed.]

Homework

• Stretching before Sleep

Practice the stretch we taught you today, in particular before going to bed. Use the handout to guide you while doing the stretches.

You can do the stretches while watching television before bed. [And you can do *salah* to improve bodily flexibility.]

• Muscle Tension Awareness and Applied Muscle Stretching

During the day, try to be aware of the tension in your body. If you notice tension in area, stretch that area. For example, you could stretch like this:

○ Straight-arm rotational stretching
  ▪ Straighten the arms until slightly tense.
  ▪ Rotate the straightened arms, once in one direction, then in the other.
  ▪ Repeat as desired with one or two arms.

○ Bent-arm rotational stretching.
  ▪ Bend one arm a little, or however much you want.
  ▪ Rotate at the wrist several times.
  ▪ Repeat as desired.

○ Finger stretch
  ▪ Straighten out and even arch the fingers of one hand.
  ▪ Wriggle the fingers.
  ▪ Repeat as desired.

○ Stretch where you feel tension [The therapist can stretch where he or she feels tension.]

○ While doing the stretching, think the following:
  ➤ "As I become more flexible in my body, may I become more flexible in my thoughts, in my emotions, may I know how to adjust to each new situation." [Or, "Oh Allah may I become more flexible in my body, may I become more flexible in my thoughts, in my emotions, may I know how to adjust to each new situation."]

- ## Head Rolling and Reassociation

  Practice head rolling. When you are at home, try to do head rolling to induce dizziness and other symptoms. Play with the sensations. It is a game.

  Reassociation during head rotation. When it makes you dizzy, think of the good times when you were dizzy:

  ❑ Rolling down a hill as child.
  ❑ Running and feeling out of breath, dizzy, and happy.
  ❑ Playing a game that made you dizzy.

- ## Practice Belly Laughing

  ### Explanation: Trying Another Emotion

  Here is another mood for you to practice, so see how it changes how you feel, and how others react to you. We call this the laughter emotion, playfulness.

  ### Prescribing Belly Laughing

  ○ Do at least two times a day, laughing from your belly.
  ○ Examine how laughing changes your mood.
  ○ Examine how laughing changes how others react to you.

  ### Modeling Belly Laughing

  Demonstrating belly laughing. This is how you do a belly laugh. [The therapist models a laugh.]

  Laughing together. Can you do that? Let us practice together, try together. [The therapist encourages the patient to follow suit as the therapist laughs, for example, making a rolling hand gesture with the hand while laughing to encourage the patient to follow suit. The therapist makes sure that the patient does a belly laugh.]

- ## Meditation Homework

  As you go home, we want you to practice the following, to practice putting your mind on a good thing, and to practice this in the following week. It is also a way to practice living in the moment with all your senses.

To Practice upon Leaving the Office: Meditation Lesson

• How the Attentional Object Determines Mood[4]

What you put your mind on will determine your mood, how you feel. Put your mind on a good object, on something that will improve your mood. For example, the Muslim religion teaches many ways to put the mind on God to enter a better state. [Here the therapist can mention: (1) *dhikr* (i.e., engaging in the remembrance of Allah), e.g., through pondering Allah's names such as The Ever Forgiving and The Most Loving; (2) *dua* (i.e., supplicating); (3) *tasbeeh* (repeating each of three distinct praises of God thirty-three or thirty-four times

---

[4] Remember to maintain a relaxed mood when teaching meditation, slowing down and deepening the voice to create a sense of relaxation.

as appropriate while using the fingers to count); (4) *salah* (ritualistic prayer), done with complete attentional focus on God (i.e., *kushoo*); (5) reciting the Quran; (6) doing *ruqyah*, e.g., by reciting Quranic verses and then gently blowing on various parts of his/her own body; and (7) doing *wudhu* (ritualistic washing) while mindful of water running down the limbs and cleansing off sins.]

• Explanation for Practicing Present-Moment Awareness (Mindfulness)

Keeping your mind on good objects. Paying attention to what is going on around you as you go home, to what is going on around you right now, such as sounds, colors, and movements, will keep your mind on good things.

Prevent your mind from floating to the past, floating to the future. By paying attention to something going on around you right now, your mind will not float to the past, to the future, to upsetting thoughts and concerns.

Not miss the beauty around you. Often we walk along, we think of this problem or that, feel angry towards something or someone, and we forget to look at the beauty of what is around us. We are thinking about this or that, feeling angry about something, are in our heads, and we walk by something beautiful, like a beautiful tree or a beautiful colored leaf, and don't even notice it. We are in our heads, in our thoughts, in our anger, and fail to notice what is going on around us. [A way to promote such sensorial awareness is by asking patients to contemplate the beauty of God's creation such as clouds, trees, and how the leaves move with the wind.]

• Leaf Mindfulness (i.e., a Form of Multisensorial Living in the Present) Paired with an Instructional Metaphor

Leaf Movement

On your way home today, notice the way the wind moves the leaves and branches. Watch how they dance in the wind. Note the way they rise and fall. [The therapist should point out the window at an example. If there are no leaves, branches can be focused on, or clouds.]

Leaves and Branches Moving in the Wind as Teaching a Lesson, as Self-Image (Metaphor): Flexibility Lesson

As you watch the leaves moving in the wind, or the branches, ask yourself to adjust flexibly to each new situation, just as the leaf (or branch) adjusts to each new current of wind.

• Mindful Eating

When you are home today pay special attention to the foods you eat. Pay full attention to their rich flavors, smells, and textures with all your senses. [Here the therapist can mention that the prophet Muhammad said "when one of you eats some food, let him say *Bismillah* (i.e., in the name of God)," and also taught his followers to praise Allah upon finishing eating; for instance, "Allah is pleased with His servant when he eats something and praises Him for it, or drinks something and praises Him for it." Can also mention that the Prophet stressed the importance of not overeating; e.g., he said, "a man does not fill any vessel worse than his stomach." The therapist may remind the patient of the overall benefits of not overeating (e.g., energy, weight loss, and reduced bodily inflammation). The therapist can mention occasional fasting (e.g., one to two times a week) as an option (i.e., if the patient is otherwise healthy and accustomed to fasting during *ramadhan*); mention that the Prophet, in addition to the month of *ramadhan,* used to fast every Monday and Thursday, and that such fasting makes the body lighter and reduces laziness. It also makes one more grateful for food (i.e., upon breaking the fast). Mention that the patient should pay special attention to (i.e., fully concentrate on) the fast-breaking foods with all the senses (e.g., their flavors, smells, and textures).]

Interoceptive Exposure II: Hyperventilation

Overview of Core Lessons

In this session, diaphragmatic breathing is taught to illustrate that normal breathing relieves anxiety, and hyperventilation is used to show that abnormal breathing can induce symptoms but that those symptoms are not dangerous. The patient is educated about breathing and educated about distress associations to and catastrophic cognitions about symptoms caused by hyperventilation and chest breathing, such as chest tightness, dizziness, cold extremities. The patient is made to hyperventilate to educate about breathing-induced symptoms, to create positive reassociations to dizziness and other sensations, to address distress associations to the symptoms, to reduce fear of the hyperventilation-induced symptoms, and to act as interoceptive exposure that creates new nonthreatening associations to the symptoms that decreases fear and other negative associations.

Outline Of Session 6

- Homework review
- Distress check (review of the Dysphoria [Anxiety/Depression] Protocol)
- Bad memory check (review of the Bad Memory Protocol [Emotion Regulation Toolbox])
- Core lessons
  1. Education about breathing
     - ➤ Two types of breathing and induced symptoms
     - ➤ Address catastrophic cognitions
     - ➤ Address distress associations

  2. Hyperventilation
     - ➤ Introduction to hyperventilation
     - ➤ Addressing catastrophic cognitions
     - ➤ Performing hyperventilation with re-association
     - ➤ Eliciting induced symptoms and addressing catastrophic cognitions and distress associations
     - ➤ Education about induced symptoms

- Stretching module for before bed
  - Behind-the-back, straight-arm stretch
  - Above-the-head, straight-arm stretch
  - Shoulder roll stretch
  - Standing, straight-leg stretch
  - Standing, bent-leg stretch

- Homework:
  - Stretching before sleep
  - Muscle-tension awareness and applied stretching
  - Practice abdominal breathing when anxious
  - Exercise
  - Practice smiling mindfulness
  - Week's meditation module

- Meditation upon returning home and during the coming week
  - Leaf-movement awareness paired to a flexibility metaphor
  - Breeze-on-skin awareness

Homework Review

Living-in-the-Moment upon Returning Home

As you went home at the end of the last session, and during the last week, did you practice living-in-the-moment, paying attention to how leaves and branches moved in the wind?

Stretching before Sleep

Last week did you practice stretching each night before going to sleep? Do you have the sheet showing the stretches, or do you need a new one?

Explore Recent Distress Episodes

Distress in the last week. Did you feel anxious, depressed, or upset at any time this last week? If so, when and why?

Self-treatment of anxiety/depression. Did you do anything that helped you when you were anxious or depressed?

Practicing the Dysphoria (Anxiety/Depression) Protocol

If you are distressed, you can do any of the following to feel better:

⟶ ***Go to Appendix C and do the Dysphoria (Anxiety/Depression) Protocol***

Bad Memory Check

- ## Explore Recent Bad Memory

Presence of Bad Memories

In the last week, did you have any recall of the past when you didn't want to, either when awake or during a nightmare? If so, please describe.[1] [If the patient had no bad memories in the last week, then ask about the most recent episode.]

Presence of Flashback

Was your recall vivid, as if it were happening again? If so, please describe.

- ## Elicitation of Self-Treatment of Bad Memories

When you had the bad memories, did you do anything to feel better?

Practicing the Bad Memory Protocol (Tools to Use upon Having Bad Memories or When Distressed)

When you have bad memories, or feel distressed, you can do any of the following. These are some tools you can use. Use whichever part you want to use:

⟶ ***Go to Appendix D and do the Bad Memory Protocol (Emotion Regulation Toolbox)***

Core Lesson 1: Education about Breathing

- ## Introducing Breathing Module

Breathing Quickly Can Cause Certain Harmless Symptoms

Today, we want to teach you about breathing such as how breathing in certain ways can cause you to have symptoms like chest tightness or cold hands, and we want to teach you that those symptoms are not dangerous.

Breathing to Relax

Today, we also want to teach you how to use breathing to relax.

- ## Education: Two Types of Breathing – Relationship to Distress

Describing Two Types of Breathing

We can breathe in two different ways:

---

[1] As described, have the patient describe the bad memories to the point of being slightly upset. If the patient is very upset, immediately start the "Bad Memory Protocol" (Appendix D).

Chest breathing. With one kind of breathing, we breathe with the bones in the chest. The bones in the chest are like the upward running wires in a bird's cage. We expand out those bones to breathe in.

"Belly breathing." Diaphragmatic, or deep belly breathing, is the other kind of breathing. It is done by expanding out a muscle that runs along the bottom of the ribcage. That muscle is like the bottom of the birdcage, but a birdcage bottom that is highly flexible. When we breathe down into the belly, the area that is like the bottom of a bird cage bows downward and the belly rises as air goes in. This is belly breathing.

Demonstrating the Two Types of Breathing

Positioning the hands. Put one hand on your belly, the other on your chest. When you breathe, notice how one or the other hand moves. [The therapist models this.]

Belly breathing. Now try to breathe slowing inward with your belly, causing the belly to rise, as you draw in air. When breathing this way, only the hand over your belly will move. Breathing this way may give a sense of relaxation. [The therapist should do a slow breath.]

Chest breathing. Now breathe with your chest, causing it to rise. Notice how only the hand on the chest moves. Notice a slight tightness in the chest. [The therapist models this.]

Belly breathing. Now breathe with your belly, causing it to rise, drawing in air. Only the hand over your belly will move. You may feel a sense of relaxation. [The therapist models this.]

Chest breathing. Now just breathe with your chest, causing it to rise. Only the hand on the chest will move.

Belly breathing. Now just breathe with your belly, causing it to rise, drawing in air. Only the hand over your belly will move. [The therapist should do a slow breath.]

Belly Breathing and Sighing: A Sense of Relief

Sigh as belly breathing. When we breathe a deep sigh of relief, we breathe from the belly, and the belly rises. This causes a sense of relaxation.

Doing a sigh. Now you try it, breathing with a sigh into your belly. [The therapist should model this, saying "ah," and showing how the belly rises.]

Chest Breathing and Fast Breathing as a Distress Reaction

When we are nervous, we tend to breathe with the chest, and also to breathe rapidly. For example, if you have children who are skipping classes, or if you have financial problems, this will make you anxious/distressed, and you may breathe from the chest, and fast.

Education about Symptoms Induced by Rapid and Chest Breathing

Symptoms caused by chest or fast breathing. Breathing from the chest, or breathing fast, may cause various symptoms:

○ feeling of shortness of breath
○ tightness and pain in the chest
○ dizziness
○ cold hands and feet
○ shakiness in the arms and legs
○ ringing in the ears
○ lightness in the body
○ feeling of numbness in the arms and legs

- ## Addressing General Catastrophic Cognitions

If you get these symptoms from breathing, there is no danger. Don't worry about those symptoms. These symptoms come from the way you are breathing. There is no danger. It is just from breathing fast and from the chest.

- ## Educating about Distress Associations: The DVD Analogy

Breathing-induced symptoms. As described, when you breathe from the chest, or breathe rapidly, it may cause various symptoms, like:

- ○ shortness of breath
- ○ cold hands and feet

Bad memories triggered by breathing-induced symptoms: DVD analogy. When you breath fast or from the chest and have these symptoms, it may cause the inner child to play a DVD from the past when you had those bodily symptoms. In this way, your breathing fast or from the chest can cause you to think of bad things from the past.

Core Lesson 2: Hyperventilation with Reassociation

- ## Introduction to Hyperventilation (Chest Breathing)

Rationale for Hyperventilation: Learning about Breathing

We want you to know which symptoms you will induce in your body if you breathe rapidly or with the chest. That way you will know if you have these symptoms again, they are just from breathing from the chest or from breathing rapidly and that there is no danger.

Breathing Fast as a Game

We will have you breath fast from the chest, to practice thinking good things when you get symptoms from breathing fast and from the chest. It is a game.

Bringing Good Images To Mind When Breathing Fast Causes You Symptoms

We want you to practice thinking of good things when you get dizzy or short of breath.

- ## Addressing Catastrophic Cognitions about Symptoms Caused by Breathing Fast

Breathing Fast Is Not Dangerous

No matter how fast you breathe, there is no danger.

Symptoms Induced by Breathing Fast Are Not Dangerous

Breathing fast may make you feel various symptoms, but there is no danger.

Learning about Harmless Symptoms

We want to show you how breathing can cause various symptoms, but there is no danger. These symptoms are just from breathing fast, breathing from the chest, and there is no danger. These harmless symptoms from breathing include:

- ○ shortness of breath
- ○ chest tightness
- ○ dizziness
- ○ mouth dryness
- ○ a racing heart
- ○ cold hands and feet
- ○ shakiness in the hands and feet
- ○ ringing in your ears

• Creating Reassociation to Hyperventilation-Induced (and to Chest-Breathing-Induced) Symptoms

Game Analogy: Breathing-Fast Game

We are now going to breathe fast from the chest. It is a game. It is the "fast-breathing/chest-breathing game."

Taking Out Good Videos: Analogy of Inner Child Watching a DVD[2]

As you get chest tightness and shortness of breath, or dizziness or other sensations, think of happy things, have the inner child pull out videos of good times when you had those bodily symptoms. As you get the bodily symptoms, as you breathe fast from the chest, think of the following:

- *Playing sports:* of when you ran fast playing soccer or swam fast, which made you short of breath and dizzy.
- *Running fast:* of playing tag, or running fast and then falling to the ground laughing, lying on your back, looking up at the clouds.
- *Riding roller coasters:* of Americans who like the thrill of riding roller coasters to become dizzy, who pay money just to get dizzy!
- *Rolling down a hill:* of when you rolled down a hill as a child and felt dizzy.
- *Playing traditional games:* of playing other games as a child that made you dizzy or short of breath such as . . .
- *Being happy to the point of dizziness:* of times you were so happy you felt short of breath and dizzy.
- *Being flexible:* of dizziness being a reminder to do the following:
  - ➢ to turn and consider all the possible roads, to be flexible, to consider all the possibilities. [The therapist should turn the head from side to side when saying this.]

• Performing Hyperventilation with Reassociation

Framing Fast Breathing as a Game

We are now going to play the "fast-breathing/chest-breathing game."

---

[2] The goal here is positive reassociation to sensations.

Naming the Symptoms and Addressing Catastrophic Cognitions

Induced symptoms. As you breathe fast, you may feel any of the following, which is normal:

- dizziness
- light-headedness
- tinnitus
- chest tightness
- a dry mouth
- tingling or numbness in the arms and legs
- shakiness

Address catastrophic cognitions. There is no danger. These symptoms do not indicate any problem in the body. [The therapist smiles, looks comfortable, like it is enjoyable.]

Encouraging reassociation. If you get dizzy, or have any other symptoms, think of games you played when young, like running or playing soccer or some other game.

Doing rapid chest breathing: Initial instructions. [It is very important that the therapist smile and seem to be having fun while doing this.]

➤ Now breathe rapidly from the chest.
➤ Breathe fast from the chest until you get dizzy, get short of breath, get other symptoms.
➤ It is the fast-breathing game!

[The patient and therapist should do rapid, chest breathing for about 30 seconds. When doing fast breathing, the therapist should smile as if it is enjoyable. The therapist should observe how quickly the patient breathes, whether there is hesitation and fear. If there is hesitation, encourage the patient to breathe more rapidly and from the chest, framing the hyperventilating, chest breathing as a game, assuring the patient it is completely safe.]

The Therapist Talks about Symptoms during Rapid Chest Breathing

➤ I feel dizzy.
➤ My mouth is dry.
➤ I feel lightheaded. [The therapist may describe any symptoms he or she feels.]
➤ You may feel the following, which is normal, and there is no danger:
  - dizziness
  - light-headedness
  - tinnitus
  - chest tightness
  - mouth numbness
  - tingling or numbness in the arms and legs

• Asking about Breathing-Induced Symptoms and Associated Distress Associations and Catastrophic Cognitions

Did Breathing Fast Make You Afraid?

If so, why? [If the patient does endorse fear, address those concerns.]

Eliciting the Induced Sensations
What sensations did you have while breathing fast?

Address Catastrophic Cognitions about the Induced Sensations
Did those sensations make you afraid?

Query about Dizziness
Did you feel dizzy? Were you afraid? Why? [If so, address catastrophic cognitions.]

Query about Bad Memories
When you were breathing fast, did any memories of the past come into your mind? If so, what memories? [If the patient has severe bad memories, consider doing the Bad Memory Protocol; see Appendix D.]

• Education about Breathing-Induced Symptoms

Distress-Caused Breathing Changes
When you are anxious/distressed, you may breathe fast from your chest.

Breathing-Caused Symptoms
This may cause the many symptoms you just felt while breathing fast.

Modifying Catastrophic Cognitions
Those symptoms are not dangerous in any way.

Reassociation
When you have those symptoms, associate them with good things.

Treatment: Slow Belly Breathing
When you have these symptoms, try to breathe slowly into your belly, holding the air in your belly for a moment before breathing out.

Week's Stretching Module with a Paired Instructional Metaphor

• Introduction to Stretching
We want to teach you how to stretch. Each week we will teach you to stretch.

• Handout of Stretching

Handout of Stretches
All the stretches are in a handout with pictures to remind you how to do the stretching. Do you still have that handout? [If not, give to the patient.]

• Rationale for Stretching

Help Sleep

It will help you to sleep by

○ helping you relax
○ preventing cramps

Flexible Body, Flexible Mind

If you are more relaxed and flexible in your body, it will help you to be more relaxed and more flexible in your emotions, mind, and ways of thinking.

Help Making You Feel Better When Upset

If you stretch when upset, it will make you feel better.

• Embodying Metaphors

While doing the stretching, think the following [the therapist can repeat this while the stretching is being done]:

➤ "As I become more flexible in my body, may I become more flexible in my thoughts, in my emotions, may I know how to adjust to each new situation." [Or, "Oh Allah may I become more flexible in my body, may I become more flexible in my thoughts, in my emotions, may I know how to adjust to each new situation."]

• Relaxing the Shoulders: Behind-the-Back, Straight-Arm Stretch

1. Stand.
2. Put the arms behind your back.
3. Grasp the hands together, the fingers interlocking.
4. Straighten the arms.
5. Keeping the arms straight, and the hands clasped, raise the arms until you feel a little tension.
6. Hold the arms there and count to ten slowly.
7. Unclasp the hands, and let the arms fall to your side.
8. Repeat one or two more times if desired.

• Relaxing the Shoulders: Above-the-Head, Straight-Arm Stretch

1. Stand.
2. Put your two arms forward and straight ahead and then grasp the hands together, the fingers interlocking.
3. Straighten the arms, producing a little tension, all the while keeping the hands clasped together.
4. Keeping the arms straight and the hands clasped together, make an upward arc by raising them upwards above the head.

5. Reach up as far as you can so that you straighten your body and spine and arms, creating a pulling feeling.
6. Keeping the arms straight and the hands clasped together, bend from one side to another, slowly, feeling the pulling tension in the arms.
7. Do this two or three times, one side and then another, all the while making sure to pull up, to reach as high as possible.
8. Unclasp the hands, and let the arms fall to your side.
9. Repeat one or two more times if desired.

• Relaxing the Shoulders: Rolling-the-Shoulders Stretch

1. Stand.
2. Roll the shoulders forward.
3. Roll the shoulders back.
4. Roll the shoulders forward.
5. Roll the shoulders back.
6. Try to tighten the stomach muscles a little as you do it.
7. Repeat two more times if desired.

• Stretching the Legs: Standing, Straight-Leg Type

1. Stand facing a wall (or a door) that has nothing on it.
2. Put both hands on the wall.
3. With the arms so positioned, the legs should be slightly apart, parallel to one another, and pointing straight to the wall. [The feet should be at a 90 degree angle to the wall.]
4. Put one leg out behind the other.
5. With that leg straight, bend the other leg.
6. Stop the bending when stretching is felt in the straight leg.
7. Hold the stretching position and count to ten slowly.
8. Now switch legs, repeating the above.
9. Both legs should be stretched this way up to three times.

• Stretching the Legs: Standing, Bent-Leg Type

1. Stand facing a wall (or a door) that has nothing on it.
2. Put both hands on the wall.
3. With the arms so positioned, the legs should be slightly apart, parallel to one another, and pointing straight to the wall. [The feet should be at a 90 degree angle to the wall.]
4. Put one leg out behind the other.
5. Bend down both legs slowly.
6. Stop the bending when stretching is felt in the calf.
7. Hold the stretching position and count to ten slowly.
8. Now switch legs, repeating the above.
9. Both legs should be stretched this way up to three times [for this session, repeat one more time].

• When to Practice Stretching

You should practice these stretches at the following times:

Practice Stretching upon Returning Home

When you get home, practice the stretching we taught you today. Do each stretch three times.

Practice Stretching Every Night before Bed

Every night, before you go to bed, for example, when you are watching television, practice the stretches we have taught you.

Practice Stretching When You Are Upset

If you do it when you are upset, it will make you feel better. [Here could mention that *salah* may also be performed to feel better such as at the various times during the day in the time windows specified in the Islamic faith (e.g., before going to bed) or when feeling upset; could mention that the patient may remain in the various physical postures (e.g., bowing and prostrating) for an extended period (e.g., several seconds to minutes), which also stretches the body to make it more flexible and relaxed.]

Homework

• Stretching before Sleep

Practice the stretch we taught you today, in particular before going to bed. Use the handout to guide you while doing the stretches.

You can do the stretches while watching television before bed. [And you can do *salah* to improve bodily flexibility.]

• Muscle Tension Awareness and Applied Muscle Stretching

During the day, try to be aware of the tension in your body. If you notice tension in any area, stretch that area. For example, you could stretch like this:[3]

○ Open the jaw, stretching it from side to side.
○ Massage the jaw.
○ Rub the forehead.
○ Rub the neck.

• Practice Abdominal Breathing When Anxious or Distressed

If you feel anxious, depressed, or upset this week, try to do the following: [The therapist should model the following.]

○ One deep abdominal breath. Breathe slowly once into your belly, causing your belly to rise.
○ With the belly fully inflated, hold it there, and count to three slowly: one, two, three.
○ Breathe out slowly.

---

[3] The therapist can stretch any place of tension. The therapist may feel tension in a certain body part owing to mirroring the patient. So the therapist should stretch that area.

- ## Exercise

Try to exercise this week. It will help you get better.

○ Take a walk.

- ## Practice Smiling (Facial-Expression Mindfulness)

Practice Having a Slight Smile

This week, try to practice having a slight smile. Practice having a slight smile whenever you meet and talk to someone. For example, have a slight smile on your face as you pass by or interact with strangers (e.g., at the grocery store or train station). Also, have a slight smile on your face when you interact with your family at home. [Here the therapist should remind the patient that the prophet Muhammad, who is the role model for all Muslims to emulate as per the Quran, where it is written that "surely there was a good example for you in the Messenger of Allah," i.e., prophet Muhammad (33:21), who was seen smiling often, and notably said that "smiling in the face of your brother is charity."]

Explanation for Why You Should Do This

Improve your own mood. This will improve your own mood.

Others will not think you are mad at them or don't like them. If you don't smile, you may frown, and others will think you are mad at them or that you don't like them.

See the Interpersonal Effects

If you smile this week, notice whether people react to you in a different way.

- ## Meditation: Multisensorial Living-in-the-Moment Homework

As you go home, we want you to practice the following in order to practice living in the moment and attending to your senses (i.e., mindfulness), to what is going on around you right now, and we want you to practice this coming week too.

To Practice Upon Leaving the Office: Meditation Lesson

- ## How the Attentional Object Determines Mood[4]

What you put your mind on will determine your mood and how you feel. Put your mind on a good object, on something that will improve your mood. For example, the Muslim religion teaches many ways to put the mind on God to enter a better state. [Here the therapist can mention: (1) *dhikr* (i.e., engaging in the remembrance of Allah), e.g., through pondering Allah's names such as The Ever Forgiving and The Most Loving; (2) *dua* (i.e., supplicating); (3) *tasbeeh* (repeating each of three distinct praises of God thirty-three or thirty-four times as appropriate while using the fingers to count); (4) *salah* (ritualistic prayer), done with complete attentional focus on God (i.e., *kushoo*); (5) reciting the Quran; (6) doing *ruqyah*, e.g., by reciting Quranic verses and then gently blowing on various parts of his/her own

---

[4] Remember to maintain a relaxed mood when teaching meditation, slowing down the pace of the voice and deepening it to create a sense of relaxation.

- ○ Drinking tea/coffee with all the senses
- ○ Wall push-ups
- ○ Pleasurable activities
- ○ Practice smiling mindfulness
- ○ Week's meditation lesson
- Meditation upon returning home and during the coming week
  - ○ Walking mindfulness with and without stomach muscle contraction
  - ○ Smiling mindfulness

Homework Review

Living in the Moment upon Returning Home

As you went home at the end of the last session, and during the last week, did you practice living in the moment, paying attention to how leaves and branches moved in the wind?

Stretching before Sleep

Last week did you practice stretching each night before going to sleep? Do you have the sheet showing the stretches, or do you need a new one?

Explore Recent Distress Episodes

Anxiety or depression in the last week. Did you feel anxious or depressed at any time this last week? If so, when and why?

Self-treatment of anxiety/depression. Did you do anything that helped you when you were anxious or depressed?

Practicing the Dysphoria (Anxious/Depressed) Protocol

If you are anxious or depressed, you can do any of the following to feel better:

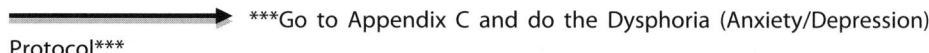 ***Go to Appendix C and do the Dysphoria (Anxiety/Depression) Protocol***

Bad Memory Check

- ## Explore Recent Bad Memories

Presence of Bad Memories

In the last week, did you have any recall of the past when you didn't want to, either when awake or during a nightmare? If so, please describe.[1] [If the patient had no bad memories in the last week, then ask about the most recent episode.]

---

[1]Through this, and the following questions, the goal is to have the patient, or a member of the group, share some bad memories. If a patient endorses bad memories, and becomes visibly upset, the patient

Presence of Flashback

Was your recall vivid, as if it were happening again? If so, please describe.

• Elicitation of Self-Treatment of Bad Memories

When you had the bad memories, did you do anything to feel better?

Practicing the Bad Memory Protocol (Tools to Use upon Having Bad Memories or When Distressed)

When you have bad memories, or feel distressed, you can do any of the following. These are some tools you can use. Use whichever part you want to use:

➡ ***Go to Appendix D and do the Bad Memory Protocol (Emotion Regulation Toolbox)***

Core Lesson 1: Exploring and Addressing Worry

• Exploring Worry and Addressing Associated Catastrophic Cognitions and Associated Bad Memories

Worry Frequency

How often in this last month did you worry to the point that you didn't feel well?

Worry Domains

What did you worry about?

Worry Controllability

Did you find it difficult to stop worrying?

Elicit Concerns about the Mental Consequences of Worry

Are you afraid that worry will damage your mind? If so, how and why? [Address the patient's concerns.]

Alleviating Concerns about the Negative Mental Consequences of Worry

Please be aware that worry will not harm you. It will not harm:

○ *Your mind.* Worry will not damage the mind.

○ *Your memory.* Worry will not permanently damage your memory. Worry may cause you to forget things more than usual, but your memory will get better when your distress gets better.

○ *Your concentration ability.* Worry will not permanently damage your ability to concentrate. It may cause you to forget things more than usual, but this will get better.

---

should be told not to recount the event at this moment, and one should begin the "Bad Memory Protocol" (Appendix D).

Worry-Induced Somatic Symptoms
- What symptoms does worry cause you?
- Did worry cause you to have a headache?
- Did worry cause you to have any of these symptoms [Here you want to determine if the patient has worry-induced panic attacks, which is common]:
  - cold hands and feet
  - tinnitus
  - chest tightness
  - palpitations
  - shortness of breath
  - dizziness or light-headedness
  - shaking hands
  - headache
  - neck pain

General Query to Elicit and Modify Concerns about the Bodily Consequences of Worry

Are you afraid that worry will damage your body? If so, how and why? [Address the patient's concerns.]

Alleviating Concerns about the Negative Bodily Consequences of Worry-Induced Somatic Symptoms

Worry may cause the following, which are not dangerous:
- cold hands and feet
- tinnitus
- chest tightness
- palpitations
- shortness of breath
- dizzy or light headed
- shaking hands
- headache
- neck pain

Explaining How Worry Causes Symptoms

Distress-caused symptoms. Worry causes these symptoms by increasing distress and fear, which causes symptoms like dizziness. But there is no danger.

Muscle tension-caused symptoms. Worry causes these symptoms by increasing muscle tension that leads to neck pain and headache among other symptoms. But there is no danger.

Explaining Worry and the Vicious Cycle

- Once worry causes a symptom, like dizziness or neck pain, you may think something is wrong with you.
- This will cause more fear, which will worsen the symptoms.

○ Then when worsening fear causes even more symptoms, you will have even more fear that something is wrong with your body.

○ This vicious cycle will continue, worsening symptoms.

Exercise Analogy to Modify Catastrophic Cognitions about Palpitations

○ Worry-caused palpitations are not dangerous. Worry may cause you to have a racing heart, and you may fear you will have a heart attack. Do not worry; those palpitations are not dangerous.

○ Palpitations as exercising the heart:

  ➤ If you exercise, if you run, it will cause your heart to go fast, but there is no danger.

  ➤ People pay money to join a gym, so they can run, lift weights, and do exercises that cause the heart to beat fast, to get the heart in shape.

  ➤ When you worry, or get scared, if your heart beats fast, you are just exercising the heart.

Do not be afraid of worry-caused symptoms. Do not worry about symptoms caused by worry. There is no danger. It is just your worrying that is causing those symptoms; there is no danger.

Eliciting and Exploring Bad Memories Triggered by Worry Episodes

Determine if worry produced bad memories. When you worry, does it cause you to recall the past?

Explore the distress associations. What distressing event did you think about? How vivid was the recall? [If the patient becomes upset, then do the Dysphoria (anxiety/depression) Protocol or Bad Memory Protocol.]

Religious Cognitive Reframing of Worry

Are you familiar with the following concepts from the Quran, which may help you to be free from worry? [Here the therapist can mention and explain the following concepts]:

• *Qadr* (i.e., divine predestination): The patient may be told that worrying will not change that which God has already decreed. According to *qadr*, worrying will not change what God has predetermined, and will therefore not alter current circumstances. The patient should be encouraged to instead engage in *dua* (supplication) to counter negative affective states; as prophet Muhammad said, "nothing can change Divine Decree except *dua* [supplication]."[2]

• *Husnu dhun bilah* (having positive thoughts about God): The patient should be encouraged to have positive expectations for the future and think positively about God (*husnu dhun bilah*), and be grateful for the present (*shukr*), irrespective of circumstance. The patient should be told that optimism about God (i.e., which indirectly affirms God's infinitely merciful nature) and displaying gratefulness for the present (*shukr*), are ways to increase one's blessings. For example, Allah says in the Quran, "If you are grateful, I will surely increase you [in blessings]" (14:7).

• *Prophetic stories* (in Arabic *qisas an-biyah*): The therapist can refer to prophetic stories in the Quran that evoke these themes. For example, prophet Jacob (in Arabic *Yacub*), prophet Joseph (in Arabic *Yusuf*) and prophet Job (in Arabic *Ayub*) are depicted in the

---

[2] See at-Tirmidhi collection.

Quran as going through major trials and tribulations. But because of their high level of gratefulness in spite of circumstance (*shukr*) and positive expectations of God (*husnu dhun bilah*), they were eventually rewarded by God. The patients may be encouraged to read the story of prophet Joseph/*Yusuf* in the Quran (chapter 12); and/or listen to lectures (e.g., on YouTube) narrating and explaining such prophetic stories.

- *Tawakkul*: This refers to putting one's trust fully in Allah (i.e., trusting in Allah's overall plan). The patient may be told that this concept is heavily evoked in the Quran; for example, "Allah loves those who put their trust in him" (3:159), and "put your trust in the All-Mighty, the Most Merciful (i.e., Allah)." Explain to the patient that the *tawakkul* mindset entails a full reliance on God regardless of circumstance, a firm conviction that God is the one who is in control of all things in the universe, and trust that God's help and assistance will eventually be granted to those who have *tawakkul* (those who rely on God).

- *Ibtilah* (trial or tribulation). The therapist can explain to the patient that the Quran mentions, "We will surely test you with something of fear and hunger and a loss of wealth and lives and fruits, but give good tidings to the patient" (2:155). This is the idea that each person will be tested by God in various ways (i.e., will inevitably go through trial and tribulation); but that trusting in God, asking God for forgiveness (i.e., repenting, in Arabic making *tauba*) and having patience, is the way to pass such tests, leading to a state of inner peace. As noted, one could mention the examples of the Islamic prophets (e.g., Abraham, Moses, Jesus, and Muhammad) who were tested by God but eventually were aided out of their troubles because of their *tawakkul* mindset. Mention here that "Allah doesn't burden a soul beyond its capacity" (Quran 2:286), that is, that God only tests us to make us stronger, but never beyond what we are able to bear. Another potent way to engender such *tawakkul* in the face of life's adversities, is to remind the patient that whenever a person goes through any hardship (e.g., poverty, loss of a loved one, sickness) sins are erased accordingly. Indeed, such adversities are a means whereby the person will be forgiven by God and become spiritually elevated (i.e., akin to the prophets); for example, the prophet Muhammad taught, "There is no calamity that befalls a Muslim but Allah expiates (sin) thereby, even a thorn that pricks him."[3] In another narration, the Prophet said (i.e., in the context of illness but with a general meaning), "No Muslim is afflicted with any harm but that Allah will remove his sins as the leaves of a tree fall down."[4]

• How to Treat and Prevent Worry Episodes

Elicit Patient's Own Self-Treatment of Worry

What do you do when you start to worry and it makes you feel bad? What do you do to treat worry and the symptoms that worry causes?

Various Tools to Self-Treat and Prevent Worry Episodes

If you want to stop worrying, or to prevent worrying, you can try any of various techniques, many of which we taught you before. The techniques are the following:

- *Stretch any area of tension* [the therapist should model stretching the arms by putting them out straight and rotating them, model stretching the shoulders by rolling them].

---

[3] Found in al-Bukhari.   [4] Found in al-Bukhari.

❑ Do stretching with visualization.
❑ You may engage in religious coping techniques:
  ➤ *Dua:* praising Allah continuously or evoking Allah's names and pondering their meanings, then asking for forgiveness or some desired end. Recommend prophetic supplications for worry and distress such as, "Oh ever Living, Oh the Self-subsisting, I seek help in Your grace"; "Oh Allah! There is no ease except that which You make easy, and indeed You, when You want, make grief and difficulties easy;"[5] and "Oh Allah, I am Your servant, son of Your servant, son of Your female servant, my forelock is in Your hand, Your command over me is forever executed and Your decree over me is just. I ask You by every Name belonging to You which You named Yourself with, or revealed in Your Book [i.e., Quran], or You taught to any of Your creation, or You have preserved in the knowledge of the unseen with You, that You make the Quran the life of my heart and the light of my breast, and a departure for my sorrow and a release for my anxiety."[6]
  ➤ *Salah:* You could tell the patient to perform *salah* during times of worry.
  ➤ Read the Quran.
  ➤ *Dhikr;* recalling Allah's names such as The Ever Forgiving or The Most Loving (Table 2). A special name of Allah to evoke in the context of worry (including anxiety and grief) is the name *Al-Khabir* (the All-Aware); the therapist should tell the patient this name is special because it denotes that Allah is aware of all your inner secrets, emotional states and pain (i.e., including past, present and future emotional states), and that He understands you, even if the whole world does not. Could relate that Allah says in another verse, "We (i.e., God) have already created man and know what his soul whispers to him, and We [i.e., God] are closer to him than [his] jugular vein" (50:16). Another complimentary name (i.e., for *Al-Khabir*), the name *Al-Latif,* which means the most kind and gentle; that is, Allah is not only intimately aware of our inner states and personal matters, but He is the most gentle and kind as well.
  ➤ *Tauba* (asking God for forgiveness) to improve worry and angst.
❑ Do the Dysphoria Protocol, which we will now review.

  ➤ ***Go to Appendix C and do the Dysphoria (Anxiety/Depression) Protocol***

❑ Live in the moment with all your senses.
❑ In order to move your mind from your worry thoughts, you can live in the moment in any of the following ways. Choose the one you wish:
  ➤ *Visual.* Look out the window and notice:
    ▪ how the leaves move in the wind
    ▪ the bark of trees
    ▪ the color of the sky and clouds, and the shape of clouds

---

[5] For a collection of prophetic supplications see Hisnul Muslim by Sa'id bin Ali Ibn Wahf Al-Qahtaani.
[6] See Ahmad collection.

- ➤ *Sounds.* Listen to sounds such as:
  - ▪ birds chirping
  - ▪ leaves rustling
  - ▪ cars passing by
  - ▪ voices of people passing by
- ➤ *Tactile.* Feel the slight air current on your face.
- ➤ *Body-movement awareness.* Be aware of the way your arms and legs move in space.
- ➤ *Breathing awareness.* Pay attention to your breath. Feel your breath as it moves in and out of your nose, as it flows in, then flows out. [The therapist should point at his or her nose while breathing]
- ❑ *Practice living in the moment while taking a walk.* Take a walk, practicing living in the moment as you walk along.
- ❑ *Engage in pleasurable living-in-the-moment experiences: tea/coffee example.* Do something you enjoy, like sipping tea or coffee, while living in the moment. As you prepare the cup of coffee or tea be mindful, and as you drink it, also mindful of the moment, enjoying all its qualities.
- ❑ *Label your emotion.* I have worry. More worry will not help me.

Good and Bad Attentional Object

Good focus: If you want to be happy, you should try to have a good "attentional focus;" put your mind on a good thing.

Bad focus. If you think of this problem and then that problem, your mind has a bad focus.

It will make you unhappy. Try to put your mind on a topic or object that makes you feel happy.

Good attentional object. Try to find a good attentional object. Switch from a bad to a good attentional object. If you think of something that makes you feel worse, it means you chose a bad attentional object. Examples of a good attentional focus are the following:

- ➤ A branch or leaves that moves in the wind, or a cloud in the sky
- ➤ Music
- ➤ A favorite television/YouTube show
- ➤ Doing exercise such as the push-ups we taught you
- ➤ Stretching your legs or another part of your body
- ➤ Talking to someone
- ➤ Enjoying tea or coffee with all your senses, as will be described.

The Amplifying Power of Attention: Pen Example

Let me give you an example of how a bad focus, bad attention, works:

- ○ *A pen in front of your eye looks huge.* If you take a pen, and then move it in front of your eye, it looks huge. [Therapist should put a pen in front of the eye.]
- ○ *Just thinking of a problem is like putting the pen in front of your eye.* This is what a problem is like if you think about it too much.

- ○ *Put the pen far away on the table and it looks small.* If you take the pen, and put it further away from you, for example, on the table, it looks small. [Therapist should put the pen on the table.]
- ○ *Put the pen even further away and it becomes tiny.* If you put it across the room, it is even smaller.
- ○ *Thinking too much about a problem is like keeping a pen in front of your eye.* If you think about a problem, and nothing else, it looms large, like taking a pencil and positioning it in front of your face. [While giving this example, the therapist picks up a pen and places it in front of the eye, illustrating this principle; the patient should be asked to do so as well.]

Channel-Changing Analogy: Refocus Attention

Let me explain this by talking about television:

- ○ *Watching certain channels makes you feel bad.* If you watch the surgery channel, or a horror movie, or a war movie, how will you feel?
- ○ *Change to a channel that makes you feel good.* If you change to a comedy, to a show about animals, or to a music channel, you will feel better.
- ○ *Tell the inner child to change channels.* When you are worrying about something, tell the inner child to change the channel.
- ○ *Too much worry does no good.* After a while, worrying does no good, it just makes you feel bad, like watching an upsetting television channel.
- ○ *Change the channel when you worry.* When you worry and it makes you feel bad, change the channel, put your mind on a different thing, go someplace else.
- ○ *Put on another channel.* Or at the least, put another channel on at the same time.
- ○ *Watch two televisions.* Watch two televisions, one playing the channel that causes you worry, the other a thing you like.

Drinking Tea/Coffee with All the Senses: Tea/coffee as the Attentional Object

Explanation for multisensorial drinking of tea/coffee. Here are two reasons to drink tea/coffee with all the senses.

- ○ *Good attentional object.* We want to show you an example of what you can do when you worry in order to feel better. We want to show you something you can put your mind on, a good thing to put your mind on. In putting your mind on just this one thing, we want you to be aware of it with all your senses.
- ○ *A way of living in the moment with all your senses.* It is another way to live-in-the-moment with all your senses.

Instructions. Make yourself some tea or coffee, and do the following. As you take the cup in your hand, note the following:

- ❏ *Weight.* The weight of the cup, a slight heaviness.
- ❏ *Smoothness.* The smoothness or roughness of the cup.
- ❏ *Temperature.* The cup's temperature.
- ❏ *Steam.* As you look down in the cup, you may notice a slight steam rising upward from the cup, twisting in the slightest breeze.
  - ➤ Ask that you be flexible like the rising steam.

- *Waves.* As you look in the cup, you may notice little waves as the liquid moves this way and that.
  - ➤ Ask that you be flexible like the waves.
- *Color.* As you look in the cup, note the color of the liquid.
- *Smell.* As you move your face closer to the cup, smell the aroma, inhaling into your nose.
- *Touch and temperature on lips.* As your lips touch the cup, note the texture of the cup and then the temperature of the liquid entering your mouth.
- *Taste.* Note the taste, maybe a little bitter, sweet, sour, or even salty.

Tea drinking as practice in multisensorial living in the moment. Attending carefully to tea or coffee drinking is a way of practicing living in the moment with all the senses.

Enjoying our senses in the now: The gift of tea and coffee. It is a way of disconnecting from your thoughts, the thoughts that circle in your mind. Drinking tea or coffee gives a chance to practice being in the moment with all your senses. So often people drink tea or coffee without enjoying all its dimensions, all its layers – what the cup looks like or how it feels, how the coffee looks visually, how it tastes or smells, its temperature. We get lost in our thoughts, forgetting the gift to all our senses that is the cup of tea or the cup of coffee.

Tea/coffee as a good attentional object: Putting your mind on tea. You are taking your tea as the object your concentration, putting your mind on something that will make you feel better, taking your mind away from worrying.

Examples of other good attentional objects. There are many good attentional objects:

- the dancing flame of a candle
- a favorite television show
- things in nature: a branch, a cloud, a flower
- the smell of perfume
- your breath as it moves in and out
- the smile of a happy child
- drinking tea/coffee with all your senses
- religious examples
  - ➤ beauty of creation: contemplating the infinite beauty and majesty of God
  - ➤ beauty of paradise: contemplating the beauty and eternal pleasures of paradise (*jannah*)
  - ➤ reasons for gratitude: pondering God's blessings and explicitly thanking Allah for these (which is a way to increase and have more of such and similar blessings);[7] e.g., the patient may make a mental list of blessings for which he/she is grateful and work these into a *dua* (supplication); such as, "oh Allah thank you from the bottom of my heart for blessing me with … " then list various blessings like: the beauty of things in one's surroundings, good health, living in a safe country with no war, loving and caring parents, beautiful and healthy children, and a loving spouse. After praising Allah and expressing gratitude, the patient then can ask Him for whatever is desired.[8]

---

[7] That is, the Quran states "if you are grateful, I will surely increase you [in blessings]" (14:7).

[8] This methodology of listing blessings for which one is grateful, and then praising God and asking for more blessings is outlined in the Quran; i.e., when the prophet Yusuf (Joseph) was victorious at the end of his struggles and brought his family to Egypt from the Holy Land, he made the following *dua* (supplication): "My Lord has made it reality [i.e., made my dream come true]. And He was

Encouraging the Use of Culturally Appropriate Treatment Techniques

When you get anxious or depressed, you should do whatever you have found useful. This may include techniques common in your culture. For example, for many Muslims, the following are helpful when distressed:

- doing *dhikr,* engaging in the remembrance of Allah, through evoking Allah's names such as The Ever Forgiving or The Most Loving (Table 2)
- making *dua* (i.e., supplicating, e.g., while evoking God's names and attributes and asking for forgiveness, and/or asking for help in any worldly matters)
- doing *tasbeeh* (repeating each of three distinct praises of God thirty-three or thirty-four times as appropriate while using the fingers to count)
- doing *salah* (ritualistic prayer), done with complete attentional focus on God (i.e., *kushoo*)
- reciting the Quran
- doing *ruqyah,* e.g., by reciting Quranic verses and then gently blowing on various parts of one's body, or reciting over a bucket of drinking or bathing water, or even over olive oil used for massaging the body
- doing *wudhu* (ritualistic washing of the face, arms, and feet) while mindful of the water that's running down the limbs and cleansing off sins

Core Lesson 2: Behavioral Activation: Encouraging Exercise Module: Wall Push-Ups

• Explanation for Why One Should Exercise
○ Exercise will make you feel better.
○ It will put your mind on a good thing.

• Examples of Exercise
○ Take a walk.
○   Wide-arms push-ups.

Here is an example of an exercise you can do. [The therapist demonstrates the following.]

1. *Starting position: Hands spread apart on wall.* Stand a few feet from the wall. Place the palms of the hands on the wall, the fingers spread out. Spread the hands and arms apart, so they are about as far out as the shoulders.
2. *Contract the stomach muscles.* Straighten the body by contracting the stomach muscles.

---

certainly good to me when He took me out of prison and brought you [i.e., my family here] from bedouin life after Satan had induced [estrangement] between me and my brothers. Indeed, my Lord is Subtle in what He wills. Indeed, it is He who is the Knowing, the Wise. My Lord, You have given me [something] of sovereignty and taught me of the interpretation of dreams. Creator of the heavens and earth, You are my protector in this world and in the Hereafter. Cause me to die a Muslim [i.e., in submission to your will] and join me with the righteous [i.e., in paradise]" (Quran: 100–101).

3. *Do push-ups.* Slowly do push-ups, making sure to keep the body straight by contracting the stomach muscles.
4. Do as many as desired, like ten or so.
5. Take a break for a few seconds.
6. Repeat.
7. Take a break for a few seconds.
8. Repeat up to three times if desired.
○ Hands-together push-up.

Here is an example of another exercise you can do. [The therapist demonstrates the following.]

1. *Starting position: Hands close together on wall.* Stand a few feet from the wall. Place the hands right next to each other on the wall with the fingers spread out.
2. *Contract the stomach muscles.* Straighten the body by contracting the stomach muscles.
3. *Do push-ups.* Slowly do push-ups, making sure to keep the body straight by contracting the stomach muscles.
4. Do as many as desired, like ten or so.
5. Take a break and stop a few seconds.
6. Repeat.
7. Take a break for a few seconds.
8. Repeat up to three times if desired.

• Alternate Days

One day, do one type of push up, for example, with the arms wide apart; and the next day, do the other type of push up, for example, with the hands next to one another.

Core Lesson 3:   Behavioral Activation: Prescribing Pleasurable Activity

• Prescribing a Pleasurable Activity

Do Something You Like Every Day

Try to do one thing each day that gives you pleasure, whatever it might be. It might be:

➢ watching your favorite TV or YouTube program
➢ taking a walk
➢ listening to music
➢ meeting with a friend
➢ going out for a fun activity

Do Something You Like Even if You Don't Want To

Even if you don't feel like it, do something you normally would like. Be active. This will make you feel better.

- ## Querying about What the Patient Does for Pleasure

Ask the patient, "What do you do to enjoy yourself, to relax?"

Week's Stretching Module with a Paired Instructional Metaphor

- ## Introduction to Stretching

We want to teach you how to stretch. Each week we will teach you to stretch.

- ## Handout of Stretching

Handout of Stretching

All the stretches are in a handout with pictures to remind you how to do the stretching. Do you still have that handout? [If not, give to the patient.]

- ## Rationale for Stretching

Help Sleep

It will help you to sleep because it

○ will help you relax
○ will prevent cramps

Flexible Body, Flexible Mind

If you are more relaxed and flexible in your body, it will help you to be more relaxed and more flexible in your emotions, mind, and ways of thinking.

Help Making You Feel Better When Upset

If you stretch when upset, it will make you feel better.

- ## Embodying Metaphors

While doing the stretching, think the following [the therapist can repeat this while the stretching is being done]:

➢ "As I become more flexible in my body, may I become more flexible in my thoughts, in my emotions, may I know how to adjust to each new situation." [Or, "Oh Allah may I become more flexible in my body, may I become more flexible in my thoughts, in my emotions, may I know how to adjust to each new situation."]

- ## Stretching the Legs: Standing, Straight-Leg Type

1. Stand facing a wall (or a door) that has nothing on it.
2. Put both hands on the wall.
3. With the arms so positioned, the legs should be slightly apart, parallel to one another, and pointing straight to the wall. [The feet should be at a 90 degree angle to the wall.]
4. Put one leg out behind the other.

5. With that leg straight, bend the other leg.
6. Stop the bending when stretching is felt in the straight leg.
7. Hold the stretching position while counting to ten slowly.
8. Now switch legs, repeating the above.
9. Both legs should be stretched this way up to three times.

• Stretching the Legs: Standing, Bent-Leg Type

1. Stand facing a wall (or a door) that has nothing on it.
2. Put both hands on the wall.
3. With the arms so positioned, the legs should be slightly apart, parallel to one another, and pointing straight to the wall. [The feet should be at a 90 degree angle to the wall.]
4. Put one leg out behind the other.
5. Bend down both legs, slowly.
6. Stop the bending when stretching is felt in the calf.
7. Hold the stretching position while counting to ten slowly.
8. Now switch legs, repeating the above.
9. Both legs should be stretched this time, up to three times [for this session, repeat one more time].

• Stretching the Legs: Sitting Type

Performing the Stretch

1. Sit down on the ground, with one leg bent, and the other crossed over it.
2. With the arm closest to the straightened leg, reach out towards the toes until there is slight tension in the leg.
3. If you reach the toes, pull back on the end of the shoe, or if you have no shoes on, pull back on the toes.
4. Hold that position, counting slowly to ten.
5. Now switch legs, bending the leg that was straight, and putting the other on top of it, straight out.
6. With the arm closest to the straightened leg, reach out towards the toes until there is slight tension in the leg.
7. If you reach the toes, pull back on the end of the shoe, or if you have no shoes on, pull back on the toes.
8. Hold that position, counting slowly to ten.
9. When at home, you may want to do it one or more times.

Sitting Stretch and Steady Improvement in Flexibility

If you practice this, you will get progressively more flexible.

Modeling a Higher Level of the Sitting Stretch

Soon you will be able to move the leg out from under the other leg, and put it to the side of the other. [The therapist models this.]

• When to Practice Stretching

You should practice these stretches at the following times:

Practice Stretching upon Returning Home

When you get home, practice the stretching we taught you today. Do each stretch three times.

Practice Stretching Every Night before Bed

Every night, before you go to bed, for example, when you are watching television, practice the stretches we have taught you.

Practice Stretching When You Are Upset

If you do it when you are upset, it will make you feel better. [Here could mention that *salah* may also be performed to feel better such as at the various times during the day in the time windows specified in the Islamic faith (e.g., before going to bed) or when feeling upset; could mention that the patient may remain in the various physical postures (e.g., bowing and prostrating) for an extended period (e.g., several seconds to minutes), which also stretches the body to make it more flexible and relaxed.]

Homework

• Stretching before Sleep

Practice the stretch we taught you today, in particular before going to bed. Use the handout to guide you while doing the stretches.

You can do the stretches while watching television before bed. [And you can do *salah* to improve bodily flexibility.]

➢ **Emphasize importance of leg stretching before bed.** It is particularly important to stretch the legs before going to bed, to help relax you, and to prevent cramps.

• Practice Drinking Tea/Coffee with All Your Senses

Practice drinking tea/coffee with all your senses, once every day. This helps you practice putting your mind on a good object.

You can practice this multisensorial awareness with any eating or drinking you do.

• Exercise: Wall Push-Ups

Try to do some exercise. Try to do the push-ups on the wall: one day, the one type; the next day, the other type.

• Prescribing Pleasurable Activity

Do something every day that gives you pleasure.

• Practice Smiling (Facial Expression Mindfulness)

Practice Having a Slight Smile

This week, try to practice having a slight smile. Practice having a slight smile whenever you meet and talk to someone. For example, have a slight smile on your face as you pass by or interact with strangers (e.g., at the grocery store or train station). Also, have a slight smile on your face when you interact with your family at home. [Here should remind the patient that the prophet Muhammad, who is the role model for all Muslims to emulate as per the Quran, where it is written that "surely there was a good example for you in the Messenger of Allah," i.e., prophet Muhammad (33:21), who was seen smiling often, and notably said that "smiling in the face of your brother is charity."]

Explanation for Why You Should Do This

Improve your own mood. This will improve your own mood.
Others will not think you are mad at them or don't like them. If you don't smile, you may frown, and others will think you are mad at them or that you don't like them.

See the Interpersonal Effects

Notice when you smile this week, whether people react to you in a different way.

• Multisensorial Living-in-the-Moment Homework

As you go home, we want you to practice the following in order to practice living in the moment and attending to your senses (i.e., mindfulness), to what is going on around you right now, and we want you to practice this in the following week too.

To Practice Upon Leaving the Office: Meditation Lesson

• How the Attentional Object Determines Mood[9]

What you put your mind on will determine your mood, and how you feel. Put your mind on a good object, on something that will improve your mood. For example, the Muslim religion teaches many ways to put the mind on God to enter a better state. [Here the therapist can mention: (1) *dhikr* (i.e., engaging in the remembrance of Allah), e.g., through pondering Allah's names such as The Ever Forgiving and The Most Loving; (2) *dua* (i.e., supplicating); (3) *tasbeeh* (repeating thirty-three times each of three distinct praises of God while using the fingers to count); (4) *salah* (ritualistic prayer), done with complete attentional focus on God (i.e., *kushoo*); (5) reciting the Quran; (6) doing *ruqyah*, e.g., by reciting Quranic verses and then gently blowing on various parts of his/her own body; and (7) doing *wudhu* (ritualistic washing) while mindful of water running down the limbs and cleansing off sins.]

---

[9] Remember to maintain a relaxed mood when teaching meditation, slowing down and deepening the voice to create a sense of relaxation.

- ## Explanation for Practicing Present-Moment Awareness (Mindfulness)

Keeping the mind on a good object. Paying attention to what is going on around you as you go home, to what is going on around you right now, such as sounds, colors, movements, will keep your mind on a good thing,

Prevent your mind from floating to the past, floating to the future. By paying attention to something going on around you right now, your mind will not float to the past, to the future, to upsetting thoughts and concerns.

Don't miss the beauty around you. Often we walk along, we think of this problem or that, feel angry towards something or someone, and we forget to look at the beauty of what is around us. We are thinking about this or that, feeling angry about something, are in our heads, and we walk by something beautiful, say a beautiful tree or a beautiful colored leaf, and don't even notice it. We are in our heads, in our thoughts, in our anger, and fail to notice what is going on around us. [A way to promote such sensorial awareness is by asking patients to contemplate the beauty of God's creation such as clouds, trees, and how the leaves move with the wind.]

- ## Walking Meditation (Kinesthetic Awareness) with Shift

As you walk home, be aware of the following:

Pay Attention to Your Walking

Leg movement. Be aware of the movement of your legs, the weight of one leg as you lift it, the feeling as it touches the ground.

Arm movement. Be aware of the swinging of your arms as you walk.

Tighten Your Stomach and Note the Shifts

As you walk along, do the following: tighten your stomach and so straighten up, and then notice how this changes the movement of your legs, the weight of one leg as you lift it, the feeling as it touches the ground, as you tighten your stomach muscles.

- ## Smiling Mindfulness

As you walk home, practice having a slight smile as you pass by someone.

[Here should remind the patient that the prophet Muhammad, who is the role model for all Muslims to emulate as per the Quran, where it is written that "surely there was a good example for you in the Messenger of Allah," i.e., prophet Muhammad (33:21), who was seen smiling often, and notably said that "smiling in the face of your brother is charity."]

Anger and Anger Protocol, and Education about Breathing and Its Use for Relaxation

Overview of Core Lessons

In this session, the patient is queried about issues of anger management, and is taught emotion regulation skills. This includes teaching the anger toolbox, a set of tools to use when angry. In this session, the patient is also taught several emotion regulation techniques; diaphragmatic breathing for relaxation, emotion distancing, and the use of adaptive emotional states. Two forms of behavioral activation are taught: encouraging exercise and doing wall push-ups and prescribing pleasurable activities. (Of note, throughout the treatment we have the patient do behavioral activation. We consider such actions as stretching and interoceptive exposure to be a form of behavioral activation in that they cause the patient to enter a new zone of experience and involve activity.)

Outline of Session 8

- Homework review
- Distress check (review of the Dysphoria [Anxiety/Depression] Protocol)
- Bad memory check (review of the Bad Memory Protocol [Emotion Regulation Toolbox])
- Core lessons
  1. Explore and educate about anger
  2. Teaching the anger protocol: The anger toolbox
  3. Breathing for relaxation
  4. Emotion distancing
  5. Practicing emotions
  6. Behavioral activation: Wall push-ups and encouraging exercise
  7. Behavioral activation: Prescribing pleasurable activities

- Stretching module for before bed
  ○ Straight-arm rotation
  ○ Standing leg
    ➢ Bent-leg type
    ➢ Straight leg type
  ○ Sitting leg
    ➢ Straight-leg type

- Homework
  ○ Stretching before sleep
  ○ Muscle tension awareness and applied stretching

- ○ Practice abdominal breathing when distressed
- ○ Practice smiling (facial expression mindfulness)
- ○ Practice belly laughing
- ○ Week's meditation module

• Meditation upon returning home and during the coming week
- ○ Cloud (sky) mindfulness
- ○ Body motion (kinesthetic) mindfulness (walking meditation)

Homework Review

Living in the Moment upon Returning Home

As you went home at the end of the last session, and during the last week, did you practice living in the moment, paying attention to how leaves and branches moved in the wind?

Stretching before Sleep

Last week did you practice stretching each night before going to sleep? Do you have the sheet showing the stretches, or do you need a new one?

Explore Recent Distress Episodes

Distress in the last week. Did you feel anxious or depressed at any time this last week? If so, when and why?

Self-treatment of anxiety/depression. Did you do anything that helped you when you were anxious or depressed?

Practicing the Dysphoria (Anxiety/Depression) Protocol

If you are anxious or depressed, you can do the following to feel better:

⟶***Go to Appendix C and do the Dysphoria (Anxiety/Depression) Protocol***

Bad Memory Check

• Explore Recent Bad Memories

Presence of Bad Memories

In the last week, did you have any recall of the past when you didn't want to, either when awake or during a nightmare? If so, please describe.[1] [If the patient had no bad memories in the last week, then ask about the most recent episode.]

---

[1] Through this, and the following questions, the goal is to have the patient, or a member of the group, share some bad memories. If a patient endorses bad memories, and becomes visibly upset, the patient should be told not to recount the event at this moment, and one should begin the "Bad Memory Protocol" (Appendix D).

Presence of Flashback

Was your recall vivid, as if it were happening again? If so, please describe.

• Elicitation of Self-Treatment of Bad Memories

When you had the bad memories, did you do anything to feel better?

Practicing the Bad Memory Protocol (Tools to Use upon Having Bad Memories or When Distressed)

When you have bad memories, or feel distressed, you can do any of the following. These are some tools you can use. Use whichever part you want to use:

➡***Go to Appendix D and do the Bad Memory Protocol (Emotion Regulation Toolbox)***

Core Lesson 1: Explore and Educate about Anger

• Frequency and Severity of Anger[2]

How angry did you get? How often did you get angry in the last month? [If the patient denies anger in the last month, ask about anger in the months before that.]

• Exploration of Causes of Anger

What caused you to be angry in the last month?[3] Please describe.

• Somatic Symptoms Induced by Anger Episode

Did you get any symptoms when you got angry? Palpitations or shortness of breath?

• Eliciting and Modifying Catastrophic Cognitions Concerning Anger-Induced Arousal

General investigation of catastrophic cognitions. Did you fear dying of heart arrest or some other problem when you got angry?

Modify the patient's catastrophic cognitions about palpitations using an exercise analogy. Anger may cause the heart to pound, but this is just exercising the heart and there is no danger.

---

[2] Use the following questions to explore the anger episodes. If the patient looks tense during the session, you can do the Dysphoria (Anxiety/Depression) Protocol, and then you can have the patient do applied stretching, attending to areas of visible muscular tension and stiffness in the patient: for example, if the patient is tightening the brow area, have the patient relax that area, massaging it as well.

[3] Of note, patients often feel anger not only towards others, but also towards themselves. Self-directed anger often results from self-blame for forgetfulness and other PTSD-related symptoms, such as not being able to work owing to such symptoms.

• Explore Bad Memories during Anger Episodes

When you get angry does it make you think of bad things that happened to you in the past? Please describe. [If the patient seems upset, do the Bad Memory Protocol; see Appendix D.]

• Educate about Anger and Bad Memories: Two-Fires Analogy

Two Fires: Past Fire and Present Fire

When you get angry, it is like there are two fires. There is the fire of your current anger and the fire of your past anger. That is, being angry may cause you to think of all the things that have made you mad in the past.

Child Example: Two Fires

○ *Child makes his mother angry.* A child may do something that makes his mother angry.
○ *Fire of past anger.* Then the mother may suddenly feel all the anger she felt about past events, like bad things her husband may have done to her.
○ *Two fires combine.* That is, the fire of the present anger may combine with the fire of past anger.

Do Not Confuse Current and Past Anger

If something makes you angry, you may be feeling the fire of past anger or may be feeling the anger you feel towards someone else. Be aware of what makes you angry right now. Do not combine current and past anger.

• Anger's Effect on Attention Allocation

One Attentional Object at a Time

You can have only one attentional object at a time. It is very hard to pay attention to more than one thing at once. That is how the mind works.

Anger Obliterates All Else

When you are angry, or when you worry about something, your mind is filled with it, you can't notice anything else going on around you, anything going on right now. Your mood is determined by what you decide to attend to and pay attention to; what you put into your mind. That thing fills your mind, and your heart, obliterating all else.

Effect of Ruminating on the Topic of your Anger

Anger obliterates everything else, obliterates what is going on around you right now. If you are angry about something, if you put your mind on what you are mad about, it is hard to notice anything else going on at that moment. If you are mad, you cannot pay attention to anything else, to what is going on around you at that moment:

Anger will make you miss good things happening. Anger will make you miss many good things that are happening.

○ *Sunset.* You may miss a beautiful sunset.
○ *How a snowflake dances in wind.* You may miss the way a snow flake dances and swirls in the wind as it floats down.

○　*Smile of a child.* You may miss the smile of a child.

You will not notice dangers: Car example. When you are angry, you may not notice dangerous things.

➤ *Angry at another driver.* For example, you might get mad at what another driver is doing, paying attention to that other driver, maybe even yelling. So all your attention is on that person, on revenge, on what they did.

➤ *Not paying attention and possibly having a car accident.* As a result, it is hard to pay attention to what you are actually doing. Maybe a child will cross the road in front of you, but you will not notice and you might hit that child. Maybe you will have a car accident, just because your heart is filled with anger and revenge, and you forget to pay attention to what is happening around you at the present moment.

• Self-Treatment of Anger

What do you do you when feeling angry to calm down and feel better?

Core Lesson 2:　Teaching the Anger Protocol: The Anger Toolbox

Whenever you are angry, you can try the following. These are some tools you can use when you are angry. Use whichever part you want to use:

➤***Go to Appendix E and do the Anger Protocol***

Core Lesson 3:　Breathing for Relaxation

• Chest Breathing and Fast Breathing as a Distress Reaction

Distress/Anxiety Causes Rapid Chest Breathing

When we are nervous, we tend to breathe with the chest, and to breathe rapidly. For example, you may think about one of your children who is not going to school, or of your financial problems. This will make you distressed/anxious, and you may breathe rapidly from the chest.

Rapid Chest Breathing Causes Symptoms

As we discussed last week, you may get many symptoms when you do rapid chest breathing like

○　a feeling of being unable to breathe
○　dizziness
○　light-headedness
○　cold hands and feet
○　shakiness

Address Catastrophic Cognitions: Running Analogy

There is no danger. In the same way, if you run fast, you will get short of breath, dizzy, light headed.

• Abdominal Breathing to Relax

If you feel distressed/anxious this week, try to do the following [The therapist should model, making sure the patient follows along.]

○ *One deep abdominal breath.* Breathe slowly once into your belly, causing your belly to rise.

○ *Count to three.* With the belly fully inflated, hold it there and count to three slowly: one, two, three.

○ *Breathe out.* Breathe out slowly.

• Deep Breathing to Relax

The main thing is to take a slow, deep breath when you feel distressed/anxious in order to relax, like a sigh.

• Living in the Moment by Attending to the Breath

Living in the Now with the Breath

You can also use your breathing to bring you into the present moment, to live in the moment with all your senses. Just watching your breathing will help you to relax. It is another way of being aware of what is going on right now in the moment around you and in your body. You are always breathing.

A Good Object of Attentional Focus: Treatment for Worry and Other Negative Thinking

You can use your breath as a way to relax. It is a way to clear your mind. When you are worrying about this or that, or when your thoughts are racing, you can just bring your attention to your breath, just watch your breath.

Paying Attention to the Breath at the Nose

❑ Just note the breath at the nose. Just pay attention to the breathing, the way the air moves in and out of your nose. [In doing the instruction, the therapist's voice should progressively slow down and become lower in tone; the breathing should become slower. The instructor can point to the nose to illustrate breathing.]

❑ Note as the air goes in through the nose.

❑ Note as the air goes out through the nose.

❑ Note as the air goes in through the nose.

❑ Note as the air goes out through the nose.

❑ Note as the air goes in through the nose.

❑ Note as the air goes out through the nose.

Core Lesson 4: Review of Emotional Distancing

• Emotional Distancing as Creating a Space of Freedom and Flexibility

Often we do things we regret if we act based on our strong emotions in the moment. Freedom is distancing from our emotions, so we can contemplate more choices. Practice the following, especially if angry or upset.

Distanced Observing

Practice just observing your emotions, not acting on them. Just watch the feeling you have: whether this is anger, sadness, or fear, just observe and let go of any emotion you experience. Just watch your emotions, not acting on them; enter a state of non-judging, of waiting and watching your emotions.

Practice Labeling Emotions and Detached and Curious Observation

- *Notice your emotion.* Be aware of your emotions.
- *Label your emotion.* Observe your mood, and label it, whether the emotion is anger, fear, worry, envy, disgust, anxiety, happiness, or excitement.
- Notice the effects of the mood on your body.
- *Cloud analogy.* Watch your thoughts and moods like you would observe clouds passing across the sky.
- *Detached and curious observation.* Just watch your mood, not acting on it, looking at it like a cloud in the sky, which will soon pass away. Observe your moods in a detached and curious observation, distance yourself from your emotion, observing it.

Emotion-as-Cloud Analogy

Like clouds in the sky, so too new thoughts and emotions will come to you. Just watch them, stay at a distance, and soon they will pass, like clouds from a sky.

Core Lesson 5: Practice Emotions

• Rationale for Practicing Various Emotions

Don't Get Stuck on Certain Emotions

Sometimes we forget to practice having different emotions. We get stuck with one emotion, like anger, envy, regret, or worry.

Lack of Emotional Range: Comparison to Cooking, Painting, and Music

You want to practice having different emotions. Otherwise, you are like:

- ❖ A painter with only one or two colors.
- ❖ A cook that uses just one or two ingredients.
- ❖ A musician who always plays the same two notes.

• Practicing Emotion Shifting: Try Practicing the Following Emotions

Here are five emotions that research has shown will help you to be happy, that you should practice. Try one. [After giving each example, the therapist should pause; the therapist should speak slowly; this gives the patient time to imagine having the emotion]:

- ➤ *Compassion. A* feeling of compassion for the suffering of all beings.
- ➤ *Joy in the joy of others. A* feeling of joy when others are successful or happy.
- ➤ *Loving kindness.* A feeling of loving kindness, a feeling of love for yourself and all beings.
- ➤ *Gratitude.* A feeling of gratitude for the beauty of nature, for those who have helped you, for the things you have.

➤ *Forgiveness.* Forgive those who have caused you any pain. [May mention here that the Quran strongly encourages forgiving others; e.g., "so forgive with gracious forgiveness" (15:85), and the Prophet said: "forgive others and Allah will forgive you"].[4]

➤ *Detached, curious observation*

    ○ *Observation and non-action.* A feeling of observing and letting go of all emotions, of just watching your emotions, of not acting on them, a feeling of non-judging, of waiting and watching your emotions. Stay distant from your emotions, in a state of curious observation.

    ○ *Label and observe effects.* Just label the emotion, look at the effects of the emotion on your thoughts and body, and let it go, stay distant from it. Say to yourself, "Oh, I have anger," and watch it, stay distant from it, let it go, not acting on it.

    ○ *Comparison of a mood to a cloud.* Like clouds in the sky, so too new thoughts and emotions will come to you. Just watch them, stay at a distance, and soon they will pass, like clouds from a sky.

Core Lesson 6: Behavioral Activation: Encouraging Exercise Module: Wall Push-Ups

• Explanation for Why One Should Exercise

○ Exercise will make you feel better.

○ It will put your mind on a good thing.

• Examples of Exercise Outside the House

○ Take a walk.

• Examples of Exercise Inside the House: Wall Push-Ups

○ Hands-apart push-up.

Here is an example of an exercise you can do in the house [The therapist demonstrates the following.]

1. *Starting position.* Stand a few feet from the wall. Place the hands on the wall, so that the arms are as wide apart or wider apart than the shoulders.
2. *Contract the stomach muscles.* Straighten the body by contracting the stomach muscles.
3. *Do push-ups.* Slowly do push-ups on the wall, making sure to keep the body straight by contracting the stomach muscles.
4. Do as many as desired, like ten or so.
5. Take a break and stop a few seconds.
6. Repeat.
7. Take a break for a few seconds.

---

[4] Narration found in Musnad Ahmad.

8. Repeat up to three times if desired.
○ Hands-together push-up.

Here is an example of another exercise you can do [The therapist demonstrates the following.]

1. *Starting position.* Stand a few feet from the wall. Place the hands on the wall, right next to each other.
2. *Contract the stomach muscles.* Straighten the body by contracting the stomach muscles.
3. *Do push-ups.* Slowly do push-ups, making sure to keep the body straight by contracting the stomach muscles.
4. Do as many as desired, like ten or so.
5. Take a break and stop a few seconds.
6. Repeat.
7. Take a break for a few seconds.
8. Repeat up to three times if desired.
○ Alternate days doing hands-apart and hands-together push-ups.

One day do one type of push up, for example, with the arms wide apart, and the next day, do the other type of push up, for example, with the hands next to one another.

Core Lesson 7: Behavioral Activation: Prescribing Pleasurable Activity

• Prescribing a Pleasurable Activity

Do Something You Like Every Day

Try to do one thing each day that gives you pleasure, whatever it might be. It might be:

➢ watching a TV or YouTube program
➢ taking a walk
➢ talking with family and friends

Do Something You Like Even if You Don't Want To

Even if you don't feel like it, do something you like. It will make you feel better.

• Querying about What the Patient Does for Pleasure

Ask the patient, "What do you do to enjoy yourself, to relax?"

Week's Stretching Module with a Paired Instructional Metaphor

• Introduction to Stretching

We want to teach you how to stretch. Each week we will teach you to stretch.

• Handout of Stretching

Handout of Stretches

All the stretches are in a handout with pictures to remind you how to do the stretching. Do you still have that handout? [If not, give to the patient.]

• Rationale for Stretching

Help Sleep

It will help you to sleep because it
- will help you relax
- will prevent cramps

Flexible Body, Flexible Mind

If you are more relaxed and flexible in your body, it will help you to be more relaxed and more flexible in your emotions, mind, and ways of thinking.

Help Make You Feel Better When Upset

If you stretch when upset, it will make you feel better.

• Embodying Metaphors

While doing the stretching, think the following [the therapist can repeat this while the stretching is being done]:

➢ "As I become more flexible in my body, may I become more flexible in my thoughts, in my emotions, may I know how to adjust to each new situation." [Or, "Oh Allah may I become more flexible in my body, may I become more flexible in my thoughts, in my emotions, may I know how to adjust to each new situation."]

• Arm Relaxation: Straight-Arm Rotation Method

1. *Straighten both arms straight ahead and bend wrists.* Straighten both arms completely straight while bending the wrists, and feel the sense of stretching.
2. *Rotate the straightened arms in one direction.* Rotate the straightened arms until you feel slight tension and hold them there a few seconds.
3. *Rotate the straightened arms in the other direction.* Rotate the straightened arms in the other direction until you feel slight tension and hold them there a few seconds.
4. *Rotate the arms back-and-forth, with the wrists bent back and fingers straightened.* With the wrist back and the fingers straightened, rotate the arms back-and-forth, feeling the sense of tension.
5. When you are tense, you can stretch both arms, or one arm, in this way. [The therapist should model the stretch with one arm.]
6. Repeat one or two more times if desired.

• Stretching the Legs: Standing, Straight-Leg Type

1. Stand facing a wall (or a door) that has nothing on it.

2. Put both hands on the wall.
3. With the arms so positioned, the legs should be slightly apart, parallel to one another, and pointing straight to the wall. [The feet should be at a 90 degree angle to the wall.]
4. Put one leg back, keeping your weight on the back leg.
5. With that leg straight, bend the other leg.
6. Stop the bending when stretching is felt in the straight leg.
7. Hold the stretching position while counting to ten slowly.
8. Now switch legs, repeating the above.
9. Both legs should be stretched this way up to three times.

• Stretching the Legs: Standing, Bent-Leg Type

1. Stand facing a wall (or a door) that has nothing on it.
2. Put both hands on the wall.
3. With the arms so positioned, the legs should be slightly apart, parallel to one another, and pointing straight to the wall. [The feet should be at about a 90 degree angle to the wall.]
4. Put one leg back behind the other, keeping your weight on the back leg.
5. Bend down both legs, slowly.
6. Stop the bending when stretching is felt in the calf.
7. Hold the stretching position while counting to ten slowly.
8. Now walk around a few steps.
9. Now switch legs, repeating the above.
10. Both legs should be stretched this time, up to three times [for this session, repeat one more time].

• Stretching the Legs: Sitting Type

1. Sit down on the ground, with one leg bent, and the other crossed over it.
2. With the arm closest to the straightened leg (though still bent), reach out towards the toes until there is slight tension in the leg.
3. If you reach the toes, pull back the end of your shoe, or if you have no shoes on, pull on your toes.
4. Hold that position, counting slowly to ten.
5. Now switch legs, bending the leg that was straight, and putting the other on top of it.
6. With the arm closest to the straightened leg (though still bent), reach out towards the toes until there is slight tension in the leg.
7. If you reach the toes, pull back the end of your shoe, or if you have no shoes on, pull back on your toes.
8. Hold that position, counting slowly to ten.
9. When at home, you may want to do this one or more times.

Sitting Stretch and Steady Improvement in Flexibility

If you practice this, you will get progressively more flexible.

Modeling a Higher Level of the Sitting Stretch

Soon you will be able to move the leg out from under the other leg, and put it to the side of the other. [The therapist models this.]

• When to Practice Stretching

You should practice these stretches at the following times:

Practice Stretching upon Returning Home

When you get home, practice the stretching we taught you today. Do each stretch three times.

Practice Stretching Every Night Before Bed

Every night before you go to bed, for example, when you are watching television, practice the stretches we have taught you.

Practice Stretching When You Are Upset

If you practice stretching when you are upset, it will make you feel better. [Here the therapist could mention that *salah* may also be performed to feel better, such as at the various times during the day in the time windows specified in the Islamic faith (e.g., before going to bed) or when feeling upset; could mention that the patient may remain in the various physical postures (e.g., bowing and prostrating) for an extended period (e.g., several seconds to minutes), which also stretches the body to make it more flexible and relaxed.]

Homework

• Stretching before Sleep

Practice the stretch we taught you today, in particular before going to bed. Use the handout to guide you while doing the stretches.

You can do the stretches while watching television before bed. [And you can do *salah* to improve bodily flexibility.]

• Muscle Tension Awareness and Applied Muscle Stretching

During the day, try to be aware of the tension in your body. If you notice tension in any area, stretch that area. For example, you could stretch like this:[5]
○ Open the jaw, stretching it from side to side.
○ Open the jaw wider, stretch from side to side.
○ Rub the jaw.

• Practice Abdominal Breathing when Distressed/Anxious

If you feel distressed/anxious this week, try to doing a belly breath. [The therapist should model the following.]

1. *Belly breath.* Breathe once into your belly, causing your belly to inflate.

---

[5] The therapist can stretch any place of tension.

2. *Hold it.* Then hold it there, counting to three slowly: one, two, three.
3. *Breathe out.* Then breathe out slowly.

• Exercise

Try to exercise this week. It will help you get better.

➤ Take a walk.
➤ Do wall push-ups.

• Practice Smiling (Facial-Expression Mindfulness)

Practice Having a Slight Smile

This week, try to practice having a slight smile. Practice having a slight smile whenever you meet and talk to someone. For example, have a slight smile on your face as you pass by or interact with strangers (e.g., at the grocery store or train station). Also, have a slight smile on your face when you interact with your family at home. [Here should remind the patient that the prophet Muhammad, who is the role model for all Muslims to emulate as per the Quran, where it is written that "surely there was a good example for you in the Messenger of Allah," i.e., prophet Muhammad (33:21), who was seen smiling often, and notably said that "smiling in the face of your brother is charity."]

Explanation for Why You Should Do This

Improve your own mood. This will improve your mood.

Others will not think you are mad at them or don't like them. If you don't smile, you may frown, and others will think you are mad at them or that you don't like them.

See the Interpersonal Effects

Notice when you smile this week, whether people react to you in a different way.

• Practice Belly Laughing

Explanation: Trying Another Emotion

Here is another mood for you to practice, so see how it changes how you feel and how others react to you.

Prescribing Belly Laughing

○ Do at least two times a day, laughing from your belly.
○ Examine how laughing changes your mood.
○ Examine how laughing changes how others react to you.

Modeling Belly Laughing

Demonstrating belly laughing. This is how you do a belly laugh. [The therapist models a laugh.]

Laughing together. Can you do that? Let us practice together. Let us try together. [The therapist encourages the patient to follow suit as the therapist laughs, for example, making a rolling hand gesture with the hand while laughing to encourage the patient to follow suit. The therapist makes sure that the patient does a belly laugh.]

• Multisensorial Living-in-the-Moment Homework

As you go home, we want you to practice the following in order to practice living in the moment and attending to your senses (i.e., mindfulness), to what is going on around you right now, and we want you to practice this in the following week too.

To Practice upon Leaving the Office: Meditation Lesson

• How the Attentional Object Determines Mood[6]

What you put your mind on will determine your mood, how you feel. Put your mind on a good object, on something that will improve your mood. For example, the Muslim religion teaches many ways to put the mind on God to enter a better state. [Here the therapist can mention: (1) *dhikr* (i.e., engaging in the remembrance of Allah), e.g., through pondering Allah's names such as The Ever Forgiving and The Most Loving; (2) *dua* (i.e., supplicating); (3) *tasbeeh* (repeating thirty-three or thirty-four times as appropriate each of three distinct praises of God while using the fingers to count); (4) *salah* (ritualistic prayer), done with complete attentional focus on God (i.e., *kushoo*); (5) reciting the Quran; (6) doing *ruqyah,* e.g., by reciting Quranic verses and then gently blowing on various parts of his/her own body; and (7) doing *wudhu* (ritualistic washing) while mindful of water running down the limbs and cleansing off sins.]

• Explanation for Practicing Present-Moment Awareness (Mindfulness)

Keeping the mind on a good object. Paying attention to what is going on around you as you go home, to what is going on around you right now, such as sounds, colors, movements, will keep your mind on a good thing.

Prevent your mind from floating to the past, floating to the future. By paying attention to something going on around you right now, your mind will not float to the past, to the future, to upsetting thoughts and concerns.

Don't miss the beauty around you. Often we walk along, we think of this problem or that, feeling angry about something or someone, and we forget to look at the beauty of what is around us. We are thinking about this or that, feeling angry about something, are in our heads, and we walk by something beautiful, like a beautiful tree or a beautiful colored leaf, and don't even notice it. We are in our heads, in our thoughts, in our anger, and fail to notice what is going on around us. [A way to promote such sensorial awareness is by asking patients to contemplate the beauty of God's creation such as clouds, trees, and how the leaves move with the wind.]

• Cloud Mindfulness

Pay attention to the clouds, how they move in the sky:

○ their color

---

[6] Remember to maintain a relaxed mood when teaching meditation, slowing and deepening the voice to create a sense of relaxation.

○ their fluffiness
○ the way they float across the sky [The therapist points at the cloud, describes it.]

• Walking Meditation (Kinesthetic Awareness) with Shift

As you walk home, be aware of the following:

Pay Attention to Your Walking

Leg movement. Be aware of the movement of your legs, the weight of one leg as you lift it, the feeling as your foot touches the ground and then lifts up again.

Arm movement. Be aware of the swinging of your arms as you walk.

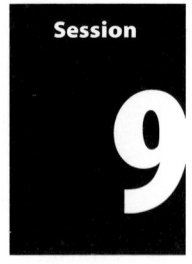

Somatic Complaints and Sleep Disturbance

Overview of Core Lessons

In this session, somatic symptoms and associated and catastrophic cognitions are explored. Sleep-related phenomena are also addressed. Victims of anxiety and depression often have these sleep-related phenomena: nightmare, sleep paralysis, and nocturnal panic. This session includes suggestions for how to reduce nightmares. Also, the patient is taught methods that help promote sleep.

Outline of Session 9

- Remind participants that this is the next-to-last session
- Homework review
- Exploring dysphoric emotion and practicing emotion protocols
  - ○ Exploring recent distressing episodes and practicing the Dysphoria (Anxiety/Depression) Protocol
  - ○ Exploring anger episodes and practicing the anger protocol

- Core lessons
  1. Exploring and treating somatic symptoms
     - ➢ Exploring somatic episodes and addressing catastrophic cognitions and distress associations
     - ➢ How to treat and prevent somatic episodes

  2. Assessing and treating nightmare
  3. Assessing and treating sleep paralysis
  4. Assessing and treating nocturnal panic
  5. How to sleep better

- Stretching module for before bed
  - ○ Standing leg
    - ➢ Straight-leg stretch
    - ➢ Bent-leg stretch

  - ○ Sitting leg
    - ➢ Straight-leg stretch

- Homework
  - ○ Stretching before sleep
  - ○ Preventing shoulder, neck, and head pain through stretching

- ○ Tea/coffee drinking with all your senses
- ○ Smiling mindfulness
- ○ Practicing belly laughter
- ○ Week's meditation module

- Meditation upon returning home and during the coming week
  - ○ Sound awareness

Next-to-Last Session

Remind Patient that This Is the Next-to-Last Session

Homework Review

Living-in-the-Moment upon Returning Home

As you went home at the end of the last session, and during the last week, did you practice living-in-the-moment, paying attention to how leaves and branches moved in the wind?

Stretching before Sleep

Last week did you practice stretching each night before going to sleep? Do you have the sheet showing the stretches, or do you need a new one?

Explore Recent Distress Episodes

Anxiety/depression in last week. Did you feel anxious or depressed at any time this week? If so, when and why?

Self-treatment of anxiety/depression. Did you do anything that helped you when you were anxious/depressed?

Practicing the Dysphoria (Anxiety/Depression) Protocol

If you are anxious or depressed, you can do the following to feel better:

⟶ ***Go to Appendix C and do the Dysphoria (Anxiety/Depression) Protocol***

Explore Recent Anger Episode

• Frequency and Severity of Anger

How often did you get angry this last week? [If the patient denies anger in the last week, ask about anger in the months before that.]

How angry did you get?

- ## Exploration of Causes of Anger[1]

What caused anger in the last week?[2] Please describe.

- ## Somatic Symptoms Induced by Anger Episode

Did you get any symptoms when you got angry? Palpitations or shortness of breath?

- ## Explore Bad Memories during Anger Episodes

When you got angry did it make you think of bad things that happened to you in the past? Please describe. [If the patient seems upset, do the Bad Memory Protocol; see Appendix D.]

- ## Self-Treatment of Anger

What do you do when angry to calm down and feel better.

Anger Protocol: The Anger Toolbox

Whenever you are angry, you can try the following. These are some tools you can use when you are angry. Use whichever part you want to use:

⟶ ***Go to Appendix E and do the Anger Protocol***

Core Lesson 1: Exploring and Treating Somatic Symptoms

- ## Exploring Somatic-Symptom-Type Distress and Associated Catastrophic Cognitions and Distress Associations

Identifying a Somatic Complaint

Bothersome somatic symptoms. Have you been greatly bothered by a somatic symptom, such as headache, dizziness, nausea, tinnitus, or by some other somatic symptom?
Most bothersome somatic symptom. Which symptom bothered you the most?

Evaluating the Somatic Symptom

- ❏ How often do you have the symptom?
- ❏ How long does it last?
- ❏ How severe is it? [In the case of headache, ask where the pain is and whether it is throbbing.]
- ❏ What causes the somatic symptom?
- ❏ Evaluating triggers
  - ▪ What is happening when the symptom starts?
  - ▪ Is it triggered by worry, anger, anxiety, or distress?

---

[1] If the patient looks tense, use applied relaxation to target areas of tension, such as the jaw or forehead, or use the Dysphoria (Anxiety/Depression) Protocol.

[2] Of note, patients often feel anger not only towards others, but also towards themselves. Self-directed anger often results from self-blame for forgetfulness and other anxious-depressive distress-related symptoms, such as not being able to work owing to such symptoms.

[It is important for the therapist to study the triggers of the symptom. Here the therapist explores the firing sequence, i.e., what the patient is doing and thinking just beforehand and when the symptom occurs.]

- Evaluating symptoms
  - When you have the symptom, do you have any other symptoms?
  - When you have the symptom, do you have any of the following symptoms?
    - palpitations
    - sweating
    - trembling or shaking
    - sensations of shortness of breath
    - feeling of choking
    - chest pain or discomfort
    - nausea or abdominal distress
    - feeling dizzy or faint
    - fear of dying
    - numbness or tingling
    - chills or hot flashes
    - fear of losing control or going crazy[3]
    - headache [In the case of headache, ask about blurry vision or flashing lights in the eyes. These may begin before or during the headache. They indicate migraine headache. Migraine headaches are common among those with distress. They are not dangerous.]
- How do you treat the symptom?

Assessing Catastrophic Cognitions about the Symptom

- Do you fear that the symptom is caused by some problem in your body? If so, what kind of problem? [Explain that symptoms are caused by anxiety or depression. In the case of migraine, assure the patient that the symptoms during the headache, such as flashing lights, blurry vision, and even temporary blindness, are not dangerous.]
- Does the symptom make you fear you may die? If so, why?

Addressing Catastrophic Cognitions about the Symptom

- Do not worry, anxiety and distress produce such symptoms; also symptoms caused by anxiety and distress are not dangerous. [Here the therapist explains how the symptom is produced by anxiety or distress.]
- Distress, anxiety and worry bring about many symptoms, but they are not dangerous. Some examples of these non-dangerous symptoms caused by distress/anxiety are the following:
  - muscle tension and soreness
  - headache
  - tinnitus (i.e., ringing in the ears)

---

[3] Another DSM-IV panic item is derealization or depersonalization but is difficult to associate in other cultural contexts so we don't add it to the list

- palpitations
- cold hands and feet
- chest tightness
- shortness of breath

◻ Vicious cycle
  - *Anxiety causes somatic symptoms.* When you are distressed and anxious it may cause somatic symptoms like palpitations or shortness of breath.
  - *Anxiety-caused symptoms give rise to fear.* Symptoms like palpitations or shortness of breath are worsened by distress and anxiety; they also make you fear that something is wrong with the body.
  - *Fear worsens somatic symptoms.* Fear then worsens symptoms like palpitations or shortness of breath.
  - *Fear-worsened symptoms cause more fear.* Soon the symptoms like palpitations and shortness of breath are made worse by fear, which then causes more concern that something is wrong with your body.
  - *Cycle of worsening.* Soon you may be very afraid.
  - *Harmless.* But these symptoms caused by anxiety and fear are not dangerous.

◻ Symptoms caused by anxiety and fear are not dangerous: Palpitations and the exercise analogy.
  - *Anxiety causes harmless symptoms like palpitations and shortness of breath.* Distress/anxiety cause the heart to go fast but there is no danger.
  - *Anxiety causes the heart to beat fast and thereby exercises the heart.* It is just like exercising the heart.
  - *People exercise to make their hearts beat faster.* People spend money to join gyms so they can exercise to make their heart rate speed up, to exercise the heart.
  - *People exercise to make the heart beat fast and to feel out of breath.* People exercise, for example running, until they are completely out of breath to exercise the heart and make it healthy.
  - *Think of palpitations as exercising the heart, and shortness of breath as exercising the lungs.*

Query about Distress Associations Associated with the Somatic Symptom

◻ Does thinking of the past or of bad things, cause you to have the symptom? If so, please describe. [If the patient becomes very upset upon asking about the distressing event, do the Dysphoria (Anxiety/Depression) Protocol (Appendix C) or the entire Bad Memory Protocol if necessary (Appendix D).]

◻ Does having the symptom trigger memories of bad things that happened to you in the past? If so, please describe. [If the patient becomes very upset upon asking about the distressing event, do the Dysphoria (Anxiety/Depression) Protocol (Appendix C) or the entire Bad Memory Protocol if necessary (Appendix D).]

• Preventing and Treating Somatic Symptoms

Prevent somatic symptoms by practicing the following:

❑ *Practice living-in-the-moment with all the senses.* Be aware of what is happening around you, and in your body, right now.
   ○ Look out the window at the branches and leaves, and watch them move slightly with each breeze.
   ○ Look at the color of the sky or the shape and color of clouds.
   ○ Drink tea or coffee using all your senses.
❑ *Do something you enjoy*
❑ *Practice muscle tension awareness* and stretch any area of tension: Be aware of any tension in your body. For example, you can:
   ➢ Relax the jaw
      ▪ Stretch the jaw, opening the mouth wide and moving the jaw from side to side.
      ▪ Massage the muscles of the jaw.

   ➢ Relax the forehead, the area between the eyebrows
      • Massage the muscles of the forehead.

   ➢ Relax the neck
      ▪ Rub the neck.
      ▪ Roll the head on the shoulders.

   ➢ Relax the arms and shoulders
      ▪ Roll the shoulders.
      ▪ Do the straight-arm rotation.

   ➢ As you do the stretching, ask that you be flexible in your body, emotions, and thoughts.

Core Lesson 2: Assessing and Treating Nightmares

• Evaluate Nightmare Frequency, Symptoms, and Associated Insomnia

Frequency in the last month. How often did you have a nightmare in the last month? [If the patient had no nightmares in the last month, evaluate the frequency over the last few months.]

Symptoms caused by nightmares. Do you have symptoms like palpitations or shortness of breath upon awakening from a nightmare?

Time to sleep again. How long did it take you to fall asleep again after the nightmare?

• Explore Nightmares' Meaning

Describe nightmare. Please describe the nightmares.
Cause. What do you think the nightmare was caused by?

• Usual Self-Treatment of Nightmares

What did you do to feel better upon awakening from a nightmare?

• Address Catastrophic Cognitions about Nightmares

Normalizing nightmares. Nightmares are related to anxious-depressive distress and will get better with treatment.

Normalizing nightmare-caused symptoms. Nightmares cause symptoms like palpitations, but symptoms like palpitations or shortness of breath caused by dreams are not dangerous.

Spiritual-related catastrophic cognitions. Nightmares do not indicate attack by a malicious spirit or that your spiritual energies are weak. [Often a nightmare may be interpreted as indicating a spirit attack or a weak spiritual status. Patients should be reminded that Islam teaches that one should ignore nightmares and avoid talking about them to others, as nightmares in essence are meaningless (have no substance and only cause unnecessary fear and worry). The patient, after a terrifying nightmare, could ask God for refuge and inner peace, and even do *salah* as the prophet Muhammad advised his followers,[4] to reduce any associated distress?][5]

• Distress Associatons to Nightmare Content

Does the dream remind you of a distressing event that you had in the past? Please describe. [If the patient becomes very upset, then one can do the Bad Memory Protocol (Appendix D) at this point.]

• Bad Memories upon Awakening

When you awoke from the nightmare, did you think of past events? If so, what bad memories did you have?

[If the patient becomes very upset, then one can do the Bad Memory Protocol (Appendix D) at this point.]

• Address Catastrophic Cognitions about Bad Memories in the Nightmare

It is normal to see bad things that happened to you in the past in a nightmare, sometimes over and over. There is nothing wrong with you.

• Nightmare Treatment Techniques

Here are some other things you can do upon having a nightmare to feel better.

Three-Screen Technique

When you awaken from a nightmare, try to figure out which earlier distressing events the nightmare reminds you of. Let me give you a television example.

○ *Nightmare television screen.* On one television screen, put on your nightmare.

---

[4] See Muslim collection.

[5] In Islamic culture, nightmares are thought to be inspired by evil spirits (*shayateen*), whereas good dreams or visions (*mubashiraat* in Arabic) are inspired by God through his angels. Narrations on the topic are available in al-Bukhari and Muslim collection. In all cases, according to the teachings of Islam, nightmares should be ignored and Muslims are encouraged not to think about their nightmares.

○ *Distress-event television screen.* On another television screen, put on distressing events that you have passed through previously that are similar to what happened in the nightmare.

○ *Day-of-event television screen.* On another television screen, put a thing that happened on the day that upset you and that may have caused the nightmare.

Transformational Technique

Change the nightmare. If you have a nightmare, then upon awakening, and during the next day, you can transform it. The event happened in the past. No need to see the image again and again. You can transform the nightmare upon awakening from it.

○ *Ant example.* For example, if in the nightmare someone attacked you, imagine that the person is transformed into an ant, then stamp your foot down on the ant.

○ *Dissolving-rain example.* Or imagine that suddenly it rains and the person or thing in the dream that scared you magically dissolves away. Change the nightmare however you want. Be creative.

Visualization Technique

You can do stretching upon awakening from a nightmare, such as relaxing the neck and shoulders and bringing to mind a good image.

➤***Go to Appendix C and do the Dysphoria (Anxiety/Depression) Protocol***

Applied Stretching

You can stretch anywhere you feel tension:

○ Stretch the arms.
  ➤ Put your arms straight out.
  ➤ Rotate your arms from side to side.
  ➤ Bend back your wrists, to increase the tension, and rotate your arms two or three times more.

○ *Stretch the legs.* Stretch your legs, using any of the techniques we have taught you. For example, you can sit on the floor and stretch your legs.

Comfort the Inner Child

Tell the inner child not to be afraid, that you are here now in [mention the country].

Living in the Now with All Your Senses

You can practice living in the moment with all your senses:

○ Look out the window and watch the leaves moving in the wind.

○ Pay attention to your breath, just noting the breath, the senses created, as it moves in and out of your nose.

Culturally specific techniques to use before going to sleep and upon awakening. [Mention the following Islamic techniques the patient may employ (see also Table 3, Introduction)]:
Before sleeping:

❖ Perform *wudhu* (ritualistic washing including the hands, face, and feet), while mindful of water running down the limbs and cleansing off sins.

❖ Pray the *witr salah* (ritualistic night prayer), the *salah* before sleep, asking God for refuge and inner peace.[6]

❖ Recite Quranic verses (chapter: 112, 113, 114; i.e., *Al-Ikhlas, Al-Falaq, Al-Nas*[7]; or chapter 2 verse 255, i.e., *Ayah Al-Kursi,* or chapter 67, i.e., *Al-Mulk.*

❖ Do *tasbeeh*: say *subhanAllah* (Glory be to God) thirty-three times, *alhamdulilah* (Praise be to God) thirty-three times, and *Allahuakbar* (God is great) thirty-four times; use fingers to do counting.

❖ Do *dhikr* of God's names (invocation of God's names and ponder their meaning), for example, through pondering Allah's names such as The Ever Forgiving and The Most Loving.

❖ Say any of the supplications (*dua*) that are narrated in the prophetic tradition and used before falling asleep, for example, "In your Name, Oh God, I die and live" (*bismika allahumma amootu wa ahya*).[8]

Upon awakening:

❖ Perform *salah-tul-subh* (the morning prayer), the morning *salah*.[9]

❖ Say any of the supplications (*duas*) that are narrated in the prophetic tradition and used upon awakening, for example, "All praise is for Allah who gave us life after death (sleep) and to Him is the resurrection" (*alhamdulillahil-ladhee ahyana ba'da maa amaatana wa ilayhin-nushoor*).[10]

Core Lesson 3: Assessing and Treating Sleep Paralysis

• Investigating for the Presence of Sleep Paralysis

Just before falling asleep, or upon awakening from sleep, do you ever have the following?

➢ *Unable to speak or move.* Upon falling asleep or upon awakening, are you suddenly unable to move even though you want to and unable to speak.

➢ *See a shape or being.* You may even see a shape move towards your body, like a shadow, or some being.

➢ *Shortness of breath.* You may feel very short of breath.

---

[6] *Witr* is an optional ritualistic prayer (or *salah*) that in the Islamic religion is performed before going to sleep at night; not to be confused with the obligatory night prayer (i.e., *isha*), which is performed prior to *witr*.

[7] The Quranic verses 112, 113, 114 are thought to bring about God's protection from devils that might harm the sleeper.

[8] For a collection of prophetic supplications, see Hisnul Muslim by Sa'id bin Ali Ibn Wahf Al-Qahtaani.

[9] *Salah-tul-subh* is a ritualistic prayer (or *salah*) that in the Islamic religion is performed early in the morning upon awakening from sleep (i.e., specifically before the sun starts rising).

[10] See Hisnul Muslim by Sa'id bin Ali Ibn Wahf Al-Qahtaani.

[If the patient doesn't have sleep paralysis, assure the patient that such events are normal, and skip to the "nocturnal panic" section.]

• Explore Sleep Paralysis Frequency and Other Characteristics

If you have such episodes, then …

○ Please describe the episode.
○ How often does it occur?
○ Did you see a shape approaching your body? If so, describe?
○ How long were you unable to move?
○ How frightened were you?

• Explore Sleep Paralysis Frequency Meaning

○ If you were frightened by the sleep paralysis, why were you afraid?
○ What do you think the sleep paralysis was caused by? [Often sleep paralysis is interpreted as indicating a spirit attack or a weak spiritual status.][11]
○ What do you think having sleep paralysis means?
○ If you saw a shape approach your body, what did you think it was? A *jinn* or *shaitan* (i.e., devil)? A *jinn* sent by a sorcerer?

• Address Catastrophic Cognitions about Sleep Paralysis

Normalize. Sleep paralysis is related to anxious-depressive distress, and will be better with treatment. It is like dreaming while awake.

Address spiritual-related fears. Sleep paralysis is not caused by a demon or other being attacking you. Sleep paralysis is sometimes interpreted as a demonic attack (i.e., a so-called "*jinn* attack") in some Muslim cultures. But sleep paralysis has a simple physiological cause, namely disruption to brain areas controlling wakefulness and sleep (e.g., could mention that sleep paralysis even occurs in animals such as mice and cats).

Address physical-related fears. Sleep paralysis is not dangerous to the health in any way.

○ It will not cause asphyxia.
○ It will not cause a heart attack.
○ It is not dangerous.

What to do during sleep paralysis. Mention that during sleep paralysis the person should remain calm and close his eyes, remind himself the episode is benign, and focus intensely on something positive (i.e., recite a Quranic verse such as chapter 2 verse 255, i.e., *Ayah Al-Kursi* or the brief chapters: 112, 113, 114; i.e., *Al-Ikhlas, Al-Falaq, Al-Nas*)], and avoid movement and just relax.[12]

---

[11] Among some Muslim populations (e.g., Egyptians), sleep paralysis is often thought to be an attack by the *Jinn* (spirit-like creatures).
[12] This therapeutic approach is called meditation-relaxation therapy for sleep paralysis.

Core Lesson 4: Assessing and Treating Nocturnal Panic

• Investigating for the Presence of Nocturnal Panic[13]

Do you sometimes awaken frightened, even though you cannot remember a dream that preceded it, but unlike in sleep paralysis, you can move?

[If not, skip to the "modifying catastrophic cognitions" section.]

• Exploring Nocturnal Panic

If you have such episodes, then …

○ How often do they occur?

○ How frightened were you?

○ Did you get symptoms such as the following:

  ▪ palpitations

  ▪ shortness of breath

  ▪ other symptoms

• Exploring Catastrophic Cognitions about Nocturnal Panic

○ What do you think causes this type of awakening?

○ If it makes you afraid, why?

○ When you awaken like this, does it make you afraid that you may die of a heart attack or some other problem?

• Modifying Catastrophic Cognitions about Nocturnal Panic

Normalizing. It is common for patients with anxiety to suddenly awaken in a panic, with palpitations and other symptoms. It is not dangerous, and poses no danger to health.

Address concerns about somatic symptoms caused by nocturnal panic symptoms. Do not be concerned about the symptoms caused by sleep paralysis like palpitations and shortness of breath. They are not dangerous.

Core Lesson 5: How to Sleep Better

Here are some things to help you sleep better; things you can do before going to sleep and upon awakening.

• Stretch before Bed

General stretching. Before going to bed, do stretching. That way when you go to bed, you will be relaxed.

Stretching the legs. It is important to stretch the legs before going to bed to prevent cramps.

---

[13] Nocturnal panic is common in patients with panic disorders and PTSD. Nocturnal panic consists of awakening from sleep and panicking, often with fears of dying of a heart arrest or some other causes, but without the awakening being caused by a nightmare. Unlike sleep paralysis, in nocturnal panic the person can move immediately upon awakening.

• Put Perfume on the Pillow

You may want to put a little perfume on the pillow, or some other scent that you like. That way you can tell the inner child, "Smell the perfume. There is no danger."

• In-Bed Breath Observation

Attend to Your Breath at the Nose

As you fall asleep, you can just pay attention to your breath; pay attention to your breath going in and out at your nose.

[When describing this, the therapist should slow the rate of speaking, to promote relaxation.]

The Reasons for Attending to the Breath at the Nose while Falling Asleep

Keep your mind off thoughts that keep you awake. Attending to your breath will keep your mind from thinking of this and that, which keeps you awake. Put your mind on your breath.

Keep your mind on the present moment. Attending to your breath will keep your mind on the present moment, on what is going on in your body, right now, at this very moment.

• In-Bed Muscle Relaxation

Contract-release relaxation. As you fall asleep, you can tighten and then let go of the tension in different parts of your body, starting with your feet or legs, such as the following:

○ Toes
  ▪ Curl your toes downward.
  ▪ Count to ten.
  ▪ Then let go of the tension.

○ Legs
  ▪ Tighten the entire leg.
  ▪ Count to ten.
  ▪ Then let go of the tension.

○ Repeat tightening/relaxation on another part of your body.

Stretching relaxation. Or you can stretch any joint where you feel tense, such as the following:

○ Rotate the outstretched arms from side to side.
○ Then rotate the wrist.

• Out-of-Bed Stretching

You can also get out of bed and do stretching, particularly of your legs, if you cannot sleep.

• Religious Methods

Muslim religious leaders (*imams*) may suggest some of the following ways to help you sleep:

Doing salah. Ask God for refuge when doing *salah* before going to bed.

Reciting the Quran. Reciting the Quran prior to sleep with the intention of gaining healing/spiritual benefits of the Quran.

Doing ruqyah. The traditional healing practice known as *ruqyah* may be recommended to patients as part of sleep preparation; for example, doing *ruqyah* by reciting Quranic verses and then gently blowing on various parts of the body, or reciting over a bucket of water used to drink or bathe in, or even over olive oil used to massage the body prior to sleep.

Listening to azhan. Finally, the patient may listen to the Quran or the call to prayer *azhan* (e.g., on YouTube), to promote overall spiritual sleep protection/improvement, and relaxation prior to sleep. Quranic recitation and the call to prayer are often described as calming and soothing, by Muslims and non-Muslims alike.

Week's Stretching Module with a Paired Instructional Metaphor

• Introduction to Stretching

We want to teach you how to stretch. Each week we will teach you to stretch.

• Handout of Stretching

Handout of Stretches

All the stretches are in a handout with pictures to remind you how to do the stretching. Do you still have that handout? [If not, give to the patient.]

• Rationale for Stretching

Helping You to Sleep

It will help you to sleep because it
○ will help you relax
○ will prevent cramps

Flexible Body, Flexible Mind

If you are more relaxed and flexible in your body, it will help you to be more relaxed and more flexible in your emotions, mind, and ways of thinking.

Help Making You Feel Better When Upset

If you stretch when upset, it will make you feel better.

• Embodying Metaphors

While doing the stretching, think the following [the therapist should repeat this while the stretching is being done]:

➢ "As I become more flexible in my body, may I become more flexible in my thoughts, in my emotions, may I know how to adjust to each new situation." [Or, "Oh Allah may I become more flexible in my body, may I become more flexible in my thoughts, in my emotions, may I know how to adjust to each new situation."]

• Stretching the Legs: Standing, Straight-Leg Type

1. Stand facing a wall (or a door) that has nothing on it.
2. Put both hands on the wall.
3. With the arms so positioned, the legs should be slightly apart, parallel to one another, and pointing straight to the wall. [The feet should be at a 90 degree angle to the wall.]
4. Put one leg out behind the other.
5. With that leg straight, bend the other leg.
6. Stop the bending when stretching is felt in the straight leg.
7. Hold the stretching position while counting to ten slowly.
8. Now switch legs, repeating the above.
9. Both legs should be stretched this way up to three times.

• Stretching the Legs: Standing, Bent-Leg Type

1. Stand facing a wall (or a door) that has nothing on it.
2. Put both hands on the wall.
3. With the arms so positioned, the legs should be slightly apart, parallel to one another, and pointing straight to the wall. [The feet should be at a 90 degree angle to the wall.]
4. Put one leg back behind the other, keeping your weight on the back leg.
5. Bend both legs slowly.
6. Stop the bending when stretching is felt in the calf.
7. Hold the stretching position while counting to ten slowly.
8. Now switch legs, repeating the above.
9. Both legs should be stretched this time up to three times [for this session, repeat one more time].

• Stretching the Legs: Sitting Type

Performing the Stretch

1. Sit down on the ground, with one leg bent, and the other crossed over it.
2. With the arm closest to the straightened leg, reach out towards the toes until there is slight tension in the leg.
3. If you reach the toes, pull back on the end of the shoe, or if you have no shoes on, on your toes.
4. Hold that position, counting slowly to ten.
5. Now switch legs, bending the leg that was straight, and putting the other on top of it, straight out.
6. With the arm closest to the straightened leg, reach out towards the toes until there is slight tension in the leg.
7. If you reach the toes, pull back on the end of the shoe, or if you have no shoes on, on your toes.
8. Hold that position, counting slowly to ten.
9. When at home, you may want to do it one or more times.

Sitting Stretch and Steady Improvement in Flexibility

If you practice this, you will get progressively more flexible.

Modeling a Higher Level of the Sitting Stretch

Soon you will be able to move the leg out from under the other leg, and put it to the side of the other. [The therapist models this.]

• When to Practice Stretching

You should practice these stretches at the following times:

Practice Stretching upon Returning Home

When you get home, practice the stretching we taught you today. Do each stretch three times.

Practice Stretching Every Night before Bed

Every night, before you go to bed, for example, when you are watching television, practice the stretches we have taught you.

Practice Stretching When You Are Upset

If you stretch when you are upset, it will make you feel better. [Here could mention that *salah* may also be performed to feel better such as at the various times during the day in the time windows specified in the Islamic faith (e.g., before going to bed) or when feeling upset; could mention that the patient may remain in the various physical postures (e.g., bowing and prostrating) for an extended period (e.g., several seconds to minutes), which also stretches the body to make it more flexible and relaxed.]

Homework

• Stretching before Sleep

Practice the stretch we taught you today, in particular before going to bed. Use the handout to guide you while doing the stretches.

You can do the stretches while watching television before bed. [And you can do *salah* to improve bodily flexibility.]

➢ *Emphasize importance of leg stretching before bed.* It is particularly important to stretch the legs before going to bed, to help relax you and to prevent cramps.

• Preventing Neck and Shoulder Soreness and Headache: Stretching

If you stretch and relax your face, neck, and shoulders a few times per day, the tension will not build up, and it will prevent body pain and headache. [The therapist should stretch the mouth, opening the mouth wide.]

• Tea/Coffee Mindfulness

Try to drink tea mindfully in the next week, every day, as described, or do some activity every day that gives you pleasure.

• Practice Smiling (Facial-Expression Mindfulness)

Practice Having a Slight Smile

This week, try to practice having a slight smile. Practice having a slight smile whenever you meet and talk to someone. For example, have a slight smile on your face as you pass by or interact with strangers (e.g., at the grocery store or train station). Also, have a slight smile on your face when you interact with your family at home. [Here the therapist should remind the patient that the prophet Muhammad, who is the role model for all Muslims to emulate as per the Quran, where it is written that "surely there was a good example for you in the Messenger of Allah," i.e., prophet Muhammad (33:21), who was seen smiling often, and notably said that "smiling in the face of your brother is charity."]

Explanation for Why You Should Do This

Improve your own mood. This will improve your mood.
Others will not think you are mad at them or don't like them. If you don't smile, you may frown, and others will think you are mad at them or that you don't like them.

See the Interpersonal Effects

Notice when you smile this week, whether people react to you in a different way.

• Practice Belly Laughing

Explanation: Trying Another Emotion

Here is another mood for you to practice, so see how it changes how you feel, and how others react to you.

Prescribing Belly Laughing

○ Do at least two times a day, laughing from your belly.
○ Examine how laughing changes your mood.
○ Examine how laughing changes how others react to you.

Modeling Belly Laughing

Demonstrating belly laughing. This is how you do a belly laugh. [The therapist models a laugh.]
Laughing together. Can you do that? Let us practice together. Let us try together. [The therapist encourages the patient to follow suit as the therapist laughs, for example, making a rolling hand gesture with the hand while laughing to encourage the patient to follow suit. The therapist makes sure that the patient does a belly laugh.]

• Multisensorial Living-in-the-Moment Homework

As you go home, we want you to practice the following in order to practice living in the moment and attending to your senses (i.e., mindfulness), to what is going on around you right now, and we want you to practice this in the following week too.

To Practice Upon Leaving the Office: Meditation Lesson

• How the Attentional Object Determines Mood[14]

What you put your mind on will determine your mood and how you feel. Put your mind on a good object, on something that will improve your mood. For example, the Muslim religion teaches many ways to put the mind on God to enter a better state. [Here the therapist can mention: (1) *dhikr* (i.e., engaging in the remembrance of Allah), e.g., through pondering Allah's names such as The Ever Forgiving and The Most Loving; (2) *dua* (i.e., supplicating); (3) *tasbeeh* (repeating each of three distinct praises of God thirty-three or thirty-four times as appropriate while using the fingers to count); (4) *salah* (ritualistic prayer), done with complete attentional focus on God (i.e., *kushoo*); (5) reciting the Quran; (6) doing *ruqyah*, e.g., by reciting Quranic verses and then gently blow on various parts of one's own body; and (7) doing *wudhu* (ritualistic washing) while mindful of water running down the limbs and cleansing off sins.]

• Explanation for Practicing Present-Moment Awareness (Mindfulness)

Keeping your mind on a good object. Paying attention to what is going on around you as you go home, to what is going on around you right now, such as sounds, colors, movements, will keep your mind on a good thing.

Prevent your mind from floating to the past, floating to the future. By paying attention to something going on around you right now, your mind will not float to the past, to the future, to upsetting thoughts and concerns.

Don't miss the beauty around you. Often we walk along, we think of this problem or that, feel angry towards something or someone, and we forget to look at the beauty of what is around us. We are thinking about this or that, feeling angry about something, are in our heads, and we walk by something beautiful, like a beautiful tree or a beautiful colored leaf, and don't even notice it. We are in our heads, in our thoughts, in our anger, and fail to notice what is going on around us. [A way to promote such sensorial awareness is by asking patients to contemplate the beauty of God's creation such as clouds, trees, and how the leaves move with the wind.]

• Sound Awareness

As you go home, be aware of any surrounding sounds, just noticing them. [As the therapist says this, the therapist should describe any ambient sounds, while pointing to his or her own ear.]

---

[14] Remember to maintain a relaxed mood when teaching meditation, slowing down and deepening the voice to create a sense of relaxation.

10

Cultural Syndromes and Ethnophysiology Related to Distress; Closing

Overview of Core Lessons

In this session, cultural syndromes are used as a means to explore catastrophic cognitions and distress associations. The session ends by encouraging the patient to do a transitional ritual. The patient is told of the next follow-up session, if that is planned.

Outline of Session 10

- Reminder that this is the last session
- Homework review
- Exploring dysphoric emotion and practicing emotion protocols
  - ○ Exploring recent distress episodes and practicing the Dysphoria (Anxiety/Depression) Protocol
  - ○ Exploring anger episodes and practising the Anger Protocol

- Core lessons
  1. Evaluating cultural syndromes and addressing associated catastrophic cognitions and distress associations
  2. Reviewing some treatment gains

- Stretching module for before bed
  - ○ Behind-the-back, straight-arm stretch
  - ○ Above-the-head, straight-arm stretch
  - ○ Shoulder-roll stretch
  - ○ Standing leg
    - ➢ Straight-leg stretch
    - ➢ Bent-leg stretch
  - ○ Sitting leg
    - ➢ Straight-leg stretch

- Homework:
  - ○ Stretching before bed
  - ○ Do a pleasurable activity like tea drinking; multisensorial tea drinking
  - ○ Emotion distancing protocol (practice labelling and distancing)

- ○ Culturally indicated transition ritual
- ○ Week's meditation module

- Meditation upon returning home and during the coming week
  - ○ Leaf-movement awareness with associated self-metaphor
  - ○ Flower concentration meditation
  - ○ Mindful eating

Announcing the End of the Treatment

Today is the last session.

Homework Review

Living in the Moment upon Returning Home

As you went home at the end of the last session, and during the last week, did you practice living in the moment, paying attention to how leaves and branches moved in the wind?

Stretching before Sleep

Last week did you practice stretching each night before going to sleep? Do you have the sheet showing the stretches, or do you need a new one?

Explore Recent Distress Episodes

Distress in the last week. Did you feel anxious or depressed at any time this last week? If so, when and why?

Self-treatment of anxiety/depression. Did you do anything that helped you when you were anxious/depressed?

Practicing the Dysphoria (Anxiety/Depression) Protocol

If you are anxious or depressed, you can do the following to feel better:

━━━━━━━━▶***Go to Appendix C and do the Dysphoria (Anxiety/Depression) Protocol***

Explore Recent Anger Episode

• Frequency and Severity of Anger

How often did you get angry this last week? [If the patient denies anger in the last week, ask about anger in the months before that.]

How angry did you get?

• Exploration of Causes of Anger[1]

What caused anger in the last week?[2] Please describe.

• Somatic Symptoms Induced by Anger Episode

Did you get any symptoms when you got angry? Palpitations or shortness of breath?

• Explore Bad Memories during Anger Episodes

When you got angry did it make you think of bad things that happened to you in the past? Please describe. [If the patient seems upset, do the Bad Memory Protocol; see Appendix D.]

• Self-Treatment of Anger

What do you do when angry to calm down and feel better?

Anger Protocol: The Anger Toolbox

Whenever you are angry, you can try the following. These are some tools you can use when you are angry. Use whichever part you want to use.

⟶ ***Go to Appendix E and do the Anger Protocol***

Core Lesson 1: Evaluating and Treating Cultural Syndromes

• Identifying Potential Cultural Syndromes

Do you fear that you have … ?

[If the patient denies having any cultural syndrome or the therapist is not acquainted with cultural syndromes in the cultural group, then ask about a somatic symptom, using the questions in the previous chapter.]

• Evaluating the Cultural Syndrome

- ❑ How often do they occur?
- ❑ How long do they last?
- ❑ What triggers the episodes? Are they triggered by worry, by anger, by something else?
- ❑ Please describe what the episodes are usually like.
- ❑ What somatic symptoms did you have during the episode?
- ❑ Do you have any of the following somatic symptoms during the episode?
  - ▪ palpitations
  - ▪ sweating

---

[1] If the patient looks tense, use applied relaxation to target areas of tension, such as the jaw or forehead, or using the Dysphoria Anxiety/Depression Protocol.

[2] Of note, patients often feel anger not only towards others, but also towards themselves. Self-directed anger often results from self-blame for forgetfulness and other PTSD-related symptoms, such as not being able to work owing to such symptoms.

- trembling or shaking
- sensations of shortness of breath
- feeling of choking
- chest pain or discomfort
- nausea or abdominal distress
- feeling dizzy or faint
- fear of dying
- numbness or tingling
- chills or hot flashes
- fear of losing control or going crazy

• Eliciting Catastrophic Cognitions about the Syndrome

- ❑ Are you afraid that the syndrome is dangerous? What are you afraid might happen?
- ❑ When you have an episode of the syndrome, does it make you afraid that something bad will happen? What are you afraid might happen?
- ❑ During episodes of the syndrome, do you fear you may die? If so, why? [Often somatic symptoms will be understood in terms of cultural ethnophysiology.]

• Addressing Catastrophic Cognitions about the Syndrome

- ❑ Do not worry, the syndrome is produced by distress and is not dangerous. You may fear you have the syndrome, but it is just caused by distress.
- ❑ Anxiety and worry bring about many symptoms, but they are not dangerous. They may cause:
    - tinnitus
    - headache
    - palpitations
    - cold hands and feet
    - chest tightness
    - shortness of breath

- ❑ Vicious cycle
    - *Anxiety and worry cause somatic symptoms.* When you are anxious, it may cause somatic symptoms like palpitations or shortness of breath.
    - *Anxiety-caused symptoms give rise to fear.* Symptoms like palpitations or shortness of breath worsened by distress/anxiety then result in fear that something is wrong with the body.
    - *Fear worsens somatic symptoms.* Fear then worsens symptoms like palpitations or shortness of breath.
    - *Fear-worsened symptoms cause more fear.* Soon the symptoms like palpitations and shortness of breath are made worse by fear, which then causes more concern that something is wrong with your body.
    - *Cycle of worsening.* Soon you may feel very afraid.
    - *Harmless.* But these symptoms caused by distress/anxiety and fear are not dangerous.

- Symptoms caused by distress/anxiety and fear are not dangerous: Palpitations and the exercise analogy.
  - Distress/anxiety causes harmless symptoms like palpitations and shortness of breath. Distress/anxiety causes the heart to go fast but there is no danger.
  - Distress/anxiety causes the heart to go fast and exercises the heart. It is just like exercising the heart.
  - People exercise to make the heart beat fast. People pay money to join gyms so they can exercise, to get their heart rates up, to exercise the heart.
  - People exercise to make the heart beat fast and to become out of breath. People exercise, sometimes running until they are completely out of breath to exercise the heart and make it healthy.
  - Think of palpitations as exercising the heart, and shortness of breath as exercising the lungs.

• Query about Distress Associations Associated with Syndrome

- Does thinking of the past or of bad things cause you to have symptoms that cause you to fear having the syndrome? If so, please describe. [If the patient becomes upset upon asking about the distressing event, do the Bad Memory Protocol (Appendix D).]
- When you have an episode of the syndrome, does it trigger memories of bad things that happened to you in the past? If so, please describe. [If the patient becomes upset upon asking about the distressing event, do the Bad Memory Protocol (Appendix D).]

• Self-Treatment of the Syndrome

What did you do to treat the syndrome, and episodes of the syndrome?

• Ways to Prevent and Treat Episodes of the Cultural Syndrome

Treat the episode practicing the following:

Do the Applied Stretching

If you fear the syndrome will occur, you can do the following to feel better:

⟶***Go to Appendix C and do the Dysphoria (Anxiety/Depression) Protocol***

- *Living in the moment with all the senses.* Be aware of what is happening around you, and in your body. Pay attention to any of the following:
  - Attend to what is happening outside, what you see outside your window, such as the movements of clouds or leaves, the color of clouds or leaves.
  - *Muscle awareness.* Be aware of any tension in your body.
    - *Muscle stretching.* Stretch any area of muscle tension. For example:
      - Stretch your arm
      - Straighten your arm, turning it side to side.
      - Bend your arm and rotate your wrist.
      - As you stretch, ask that you be flexible in your body and mind.

Core Lesson 2: Reviewing Some Key Lessons Learned in Treatment

• Summarizing: Skills Learned (Stretching, Distancing from Mood, Being More Flexible in Body and Mind)

○ We have tried to teach you some skills, like the following:

➤ How to use stretching and good images when you are distressed or anxious. [The therapist should demonstrate this by tightening the stomach muscles, lifting the shoulders, dropping them, and rotating the head.]

➤ How to use other emotions like loving kindness.

➤ How to live in the moment with all your senses, like paying attention to the motion of leaves in the wind or clouds in the sky.

➤ How to stretch your legs before going to bed, to prevent cramps.

➤ How to distance yourself from your emotions, so that you can consider other ways of acting and feeling, so you can be more flexible in your life and relationships, in your way of thinking.

Week's Stretching Module with a Paired Instructional Metaphor

• Introduction to Stretching

We taught you during the previous sessions how to stretch.

• Handout of Stretching

Handout of Stretches

All the stretches are in a handout with pictures to remind you how to do the stretching. Do you still have that handout?

• Rationale for Stretching

Help with Sleeping

It will help you to sleep because it

○ will help you relax

○ will prevent cramps

Flexible Body, Flexible Mind

If you are more relaxed and flexible in your body, you will be more relaxed and more flexible in your emotions, mind, and ways of thinking.

Help Make You Feel Better When Upset

If you stretch when upset, it will make you feel better.

- ## Embodying Metaphors

While doing the stretching, think of the following [the therapist should repeat this self-statement while the actual stretching is being done]:

➢ "As I become more flexible in my body, may I become more flexible in my thoughts, in my emotions, may I know how to adjust to each new situation." [Or, "Oh Allah may I become more flexible in my body, may I become more flexible in my thoughts, in my emotions, may I know how to adjust to each new situation."]

- ## Relaxing the Shoulders: Behind-the-Back, Straight-Arm Stretch

1. Stand.
2. Put the arms behind your back.
3. Grasp the hands together, the fingers interlocking.
4. Straighten the arms.
5. Keeping the arms straight, and the hands clasped, raise the arms until you feel a little tension.
6. Hold the arms there and count to ten slowly.
7. Unclasp the hands, and let the arms fall to your side.
8. Repeat one or two more times if desired.

- ## Relaxing the Shoulders: Above-the-Head, Straight-Arm Stretch

1. Stand.
2. Put your two arms forward and straight ahead and then grasp the hands together, the fingers interlocking.
3. Straighten the arms, producing a little tension, all the while keeping the hands clasped together.
4. Keeping the arms straight and the hands clasped together, make an upward arc by raising them upwards above the head.
5. Reach up as far as you can so that you straighten your body and spine and arms, creating a pulling feeling.
6. Keeping the arms straight and the hands clasped together, bend from one side to another, slowly, feeling the pulling tension in the arms.
7. Do this two or three times, one side and then another, all the while making sure to pull up, to reach as high as possible.
8. Unclasp the hands, and let the arms fall to your side.
9. Repeat one or two more times if desired.

- ## Relaxing the Shoulders: Rolling-the-Shoulders Stretch

1. Stand.
2. Roll the shoulders forward.
3. Roll the shoulders back.
4. Roll the shoulders forward.

5. Roll the shoulders back.
6. Try to tighten the stomach muscles a little as you do it.
7. Repeat one or two more times if desired.

• Stretching the Legs: Standing, Straight-Leg Type

1. Stand facing a wall (or a door) that has nothing on it.
2. Put both hands on the wall.
3. With the arms so positioned, the legs should be slightly apart, parallel to one another, and pointing straight to the wall. [The feet should be at a 90 degree angle to the wall.]
4. Put one leg out behind the other.
5. With that leg straight, bend the other leg.
6. Stop the bending when stretching is felt in the straight leg.
7. Hold the stretching position while counting to ten slowly.
8. Now switch legs, repeating the above.
9. Both legs should be stretched this way up to three times.

• Stretching the Legs: Standing, Bent-Leg Type

1. Stand facing a wall (or a door) that has nothing on it.
2. Put both hands on the wall.
3. With the arms so positioned, the legs should be slightly apart, parallel to one another, and pointing straight to the wall. [The feet should be at a 90-degree angle to the wall.]
4. Put one leg out behind the other.
5. Bend down both legs, slowly.
6. Stop the bending when stretching is felt in the calf.
7. Hold the stretching position while counting to ten slowly.
8. Now switch legs, repeating the above.
9. Both legs should be stretched this time up to three times [for this session, repeat one more time].

• Stretching the Legs: Sitting Type

Performing the Stretch

1. Sit down on the ground, with one leg bent, and the other crossed over it.
2. With the arm closest to the straightened leg, reach out towards the toes until there is slight tension in the leg.
3. If you reach the toes, pull back on the end of the shoe, or if you have no shoes on, on your toes.
4. Hold that position, counting slowly to ten.
5. Now switch legs, bending the leg that was straight, and putting the other on top of it, straight out.
6. With the arm closest to the straightened leg, reach out towards the toes until there is slight tension in the leg.
7. If you reach the toes, pull back on the end of the shoe, or if you have no shoes on, on your toes.

8. Hold that position, counting slowly to ten.
9. When at home, you may want to do it one or more times.

Sitting Stretch and Steady Improvement in Flexibility
If you practice this, you will get progressively more flexible.

Modeling a Higher Level of the Sitting Stretch
Soon you will be able to move the leg out from under the other leg, and put it to the side of the other. [The therapist models this.]

• When to Practice Stretching
You should practice these stretches at the following times:

Practice Stretching upon Returning Home
When you get home, practice the stretching we taught you today. Do each stretch three times.

Practice Stretching Every Night Before Bed
Every night, before you go to bed, for example, when you are watching television, practice the stretches we have taught you.

Practice Stretching When You Are Upset
If you practice stretching when you are upset, it will make you feel better. [Here the therapist could mention that *salah* may also be performed to feel better such as at the various times during the day in the time windows specified in the Islamic faith (e.g., before going to bed) or when feeling upset; could mention that the patient may remain in the various physical postures (e.g., bowing and prostrating) for an extended period (e.g., several seconds to minutes), which also stretches the body to make it more flexible and relaxed.]

Homework
• Stretching before Sleep
Practice the stretch we taught you today, in particular before going to bed. Use the handout to guide you while doing the stretches.

You can do the stretches while watching television before bed. [And you can do *salah* to improve bodily flexibility.]

➤ *Emphasize importance of leg stretching before bed.* It is particularly important to stretch the legs before going to bed, to help relax you and to prevent cramps.

• Do a Pleasurable Activity Like Drinking Tea or Coffee Using All Your Senses
Try to drink tea/coffee every day in the next week, as described, or do some activity every day that gives you pleasure.

• Practice Labelling Emotions and Detached and Curious Observation

- ❑ *Notice your emotion.* Be aware of your emotions.
- ❑ *Label your emotion.* Observe your mood and label it, whether the emotion is anger, fear, worry, envy, disgust, anxiety, happiness, or excitement.
- ❑ *Notice the effects of the mood on your body.*
- ❑ *Cloud analogy.* Watch your thoughts and moods like you would observe clouds passing across the sky.
- ❑ *Detached and curious observation.* Just watch your mood, not acting on it, looking at it like a cloud in the sky, which will soon pass away. Observe your moods in a detached and curious observation, distancing yourself from your emotion, observing it.

• Culturally Indicated Ritual of Purification or Transition

Now that you have finished the treatment, we want you to do something to mark the end, the fact that you have completed the treatment. You can do something special to mark the end and celebrate. [The therapist may recommend doing *wudhu* (ritualistic washing of the face, arms, and feet). The patient should be reminded that during *wudhu* any body part that comes in contact with water is cleansed of sin; for instance, by rinsing the mouth it is cleansed from any sins, such as from profanities uttered during the course of the day. And it should be stressed that Muslims are encouraged to be mindful of God during *wudhu*; on bodily cleansing, such as water running down the limbs and cleansing off sins. The patient should be told that *wudhu* is a way to transform into a more spiritually clean state. Even greater than *wudhu* is the act of *ghusl*[3] (i.e., ritualistic washing of the entire body). The patient should therefore ideally be encouraged to perform *ghusl*; remind the patient that *ghusl* is usually performed before going to the mosque on Fridays or religious festivities (i.e., *eid*), and also after religious conversion; it thus represents entering into a more clean spiritual state.]

• Multisensorial Living-in-the-Moment Homework

Also, we want you to practice the following type of multisensorial living in the moment when you go home today, and in the following week.

To Practice Upon Leaving the Office: Meditation Lesson

• How the Attentional Object Determines Mood[4]

What you put your mind on will determine your mood and how you feel. Put your mind on a good object, on something that will improve your mood. For example, the Muslim religion

---

[3] *Ghusl* is a greater and more extensive form of spiritual and physical purification. It is performed after sexual intercourse (i.e., prior to *salah*), after menstrual periods for women, and ideally before going to the mosque on Fridays or for religious festivities, and also after religious conversion.

[4] Remember to maintain a relaxed mood when teaching meditation, slowing down the pace of the voice and deepening it to create a sense of relaxation.

teaches many ways to put the mind on God to enter a better state. [Here the therapist can mention: (1) *dhikr* (i.e., engaging in the remembrance of Allah), e.g., through pondering Allah's names such as The Ever Forgiving and The Most Loving; (2) *dua* (i.e., supplicating); (3) *tasbeeh* (repeating each of three distinct praises of God thirty-three or thirty-four times as appropriate while using the fingers to count); (4) *salah* (ritualistic prayer), done with complete attentional focus on God (i.e., *kushoo*); (5) reciting the Quran; (6) doing *ruqyah*, e.g., by reciting Quranic verses and then gently blowing on various parts of his/her own body; and (7) doing *wudhu* (ritualistic washing) while mindful of water running down the limbs and cleansing off sins.]

• Explanation for Practicing Present-Moment Awareness (Mindfulness)

Keeping your mind on a good object. Paying attention to what is going on around you as you go home and to what is going on around you right now, such as sounds, colors, movements, will keep your mind on a good thing.

Prevent your mind from floating to the past, floating to the future. By paying attention to something going on around you right now, your mind will not float to the past, to the future, or to upsetting thoughts and concerns.

Don't miss the beauty around you. Often we walk along, we think of this problem or that, feel angry towards something or someone, and we forget to look at the beauty of what is around us. We are thinking about this or that, feeling angry about something, are in our heads, and we walk by something beautiful, like a beautiful tree or a beautiful colored leaf, and don't even notice it. We are in our heads, in our thoughts, in our anger, and fail to notice what is going on around us. [A way to promote such sensorial awareness is by asking patients to contemplate the beauty of God's creation such as clouds, trees, and how the leaves move with the wind.]

• Leaf Mindfulness

On your way home today, we want you to notice:

Leaf Movement

Notice how the wind moves the leaves, and branches. Watch how they dance in the wind. Note the way they rise and fall. [The therapist should point out the window at an example. If there are no leaves, branches can be focused on, or clouds.]

Wind-Moved Leaves and Branches as Teaching a Lesson, as Self-Image (Metaphor): Flexibility Lesson

As you watch the leaves or the branches moving in the wind, ask that you can flexibly adjust to each new situation, just as the leaf (or branch) adjusts to each new current of wind.

• Flower Concentration Meditation

Pick a flower on the way home, and put it in a container when you get there. Meditate on the image and keep that image in your mind. [If a flower is not available, use a leaf or small branch, maybe one with berries or seedpods.]

• Mindful Eating

When you are home today pay special attention to the foods you eat. Pay full attention to their rich flavors, smells, and textures with all your senses. [Here the therapist can mention that the prophet Muhammad said that "when one of you eats some food, let him say *Bismillah* (i.e., in the name of God)," and also taught his followers to praise Allah upon finishing eating; for instance, "Allah is pleased with His servant when he eats something and praises Him for it, or drinks something and praises Him for it." Can also mention that the Prophet stressed the importance of not overeating; e.g., he said, "a man does not fill any vessel worse than his stomach." The therapist may remind the patient of the overall benefits of not overeating (e.g., energy, weight loss, and reduced bodily inflammation). The therapist can mention occasional fasting (e.g., one to two times a week) as an option (i.e., if the patient is otherwise healthy and accustomed to fasting during *ramadhan*); mention that the Prophet, in addition to the month of *ramadhan,* used to fast every Monday and Thursday, and that such fasting makes the body lighter and reduces laziness. It also makes one more grateful for food (i.e., upon breaking the fast). Mention that the patient should pay special attention to (i.e., fully concentrate on) the fast-breaking foods with all the senses (e.g., their flavors, smells, and textures).]

Appendices

Appendix A Stretching Handout

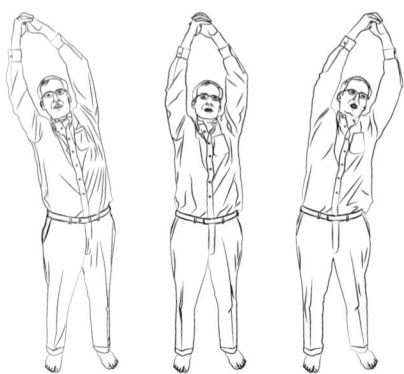

Above-the-head straight-arm stretch

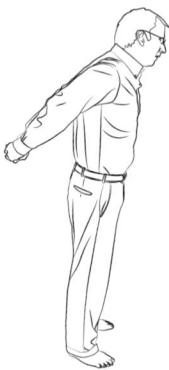

Behind-the-back straight-arm stretch

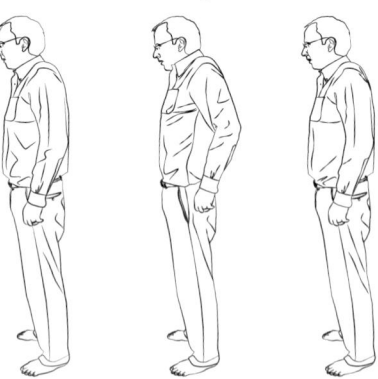

Shoulder roll stretch

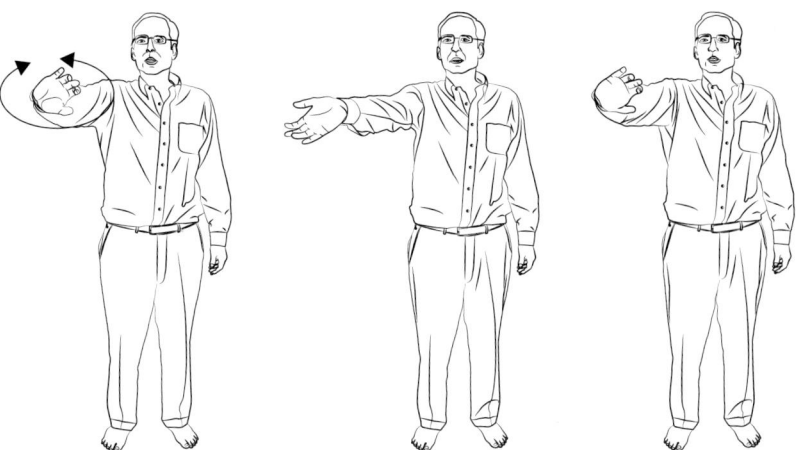

Straight-arm rotational stretch

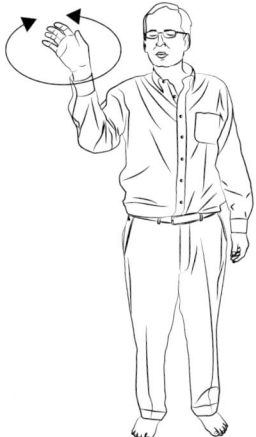

Bent-arm wrist rotational stretch

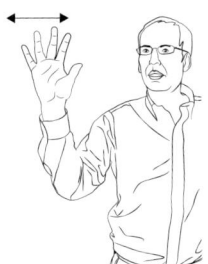

Finger stretch

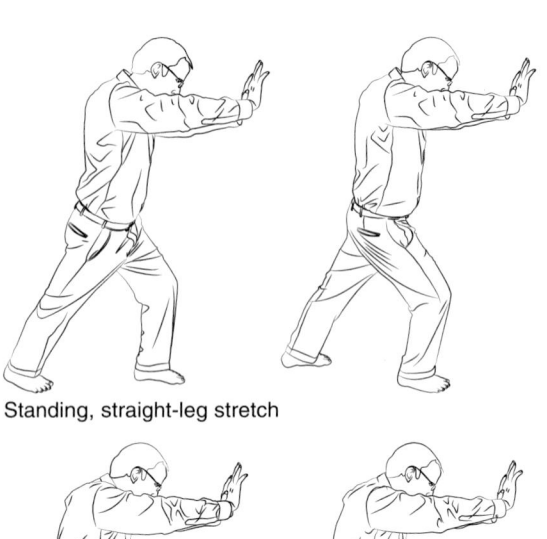

Standing, straight-leg stretch

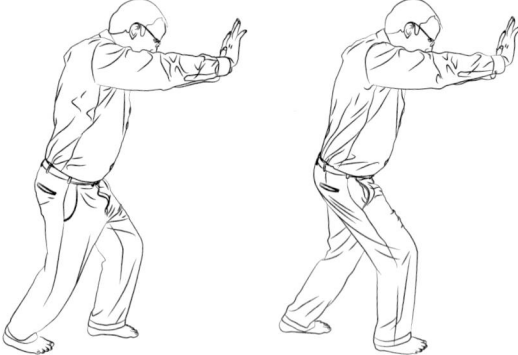

Standing, bent-leg stretch

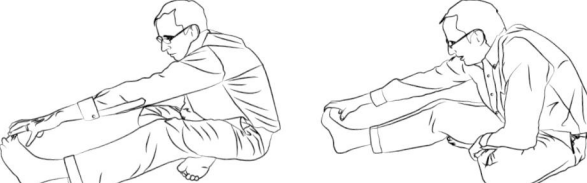

Sitting, basic leg stretch

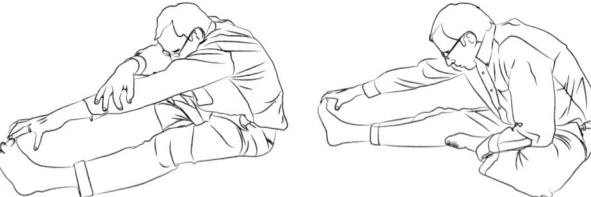

Sitting, advanced leg stretch

Appendix B Toe-to-Head Relaxation with Visualization

We want to teach you one way to relax the entire body. When you are asked to relax a particular muscle, after releasing the tension, feel free to stretch that muscle, or any other muscle that is tense.

- **Addressing catastrophic cognitions about rotations at the joints, especially the neck**

Rotating joints isn't dangerous

When you do rotations at the joints, including rotations of the neck, it is not dangerous.

Sounds from muscles do not indicate problems

If you hear any sounds as you rotate the head, there is no danger. It is just the sound of relaxing your muscles and tendons. The sounds have nothing to do with blood vessels, blood pressure, or any other problems, and these motions will cause no damage.[1]

Safe even if you have high blood pressure

Even if you have high blood pressure, rotating the head is not dangerous.

- **Decreasing anxiety about learning the toe-to-head relaxation procedure: Bicycle analogy**

You will now learn how to relax your muscles, by tensing them and letting go of the tension and then stretching them.

Bicycle analogy

If you don't remember everything, that is fine. It is like riding a bicycle. At first you may not be able to do it perfectly, but soon it will be easy.

- **Teaching your whole body muscular relaxation**

We will now teach you how to relax your muscles by tightening them, releasing them, and then stretching them.

[During the following, the patient ideally should sit in a comfortable chair, closing the eyes most of the time, periodically opening them to see the therapist's modeling of the stretching.]

❑ *Feet and legs.* Now let us relax and stretch the feet and legs.

1. *Tighten.* Curl the toes of both feet downward in your shoes; at the same time push down the tips of your feet toward the ground; while doing this, tighten the muscles in your calves and thighs.

2. *Count.* Now hold this position as you count slowly to ten: one, two, three, four, five, six, seven, eight, nine, ten. [Therapist counts slowly, with a calm, deep voice, allowing about a second for each number, about the time it would take to count "one one thousand."]

3. *Release.* Now let go of the tension.

4. *Positive imagery.* Notice the feeling of warmth in your feet, the release of tension.

5. *Stretch the muscle.* To stretch and relax these same muscles, try wiggling the toes, rotating at the ankle.

6. *Stretch any area of tension.* Wherever you feel tense in your body, do stretching; for example, by rolling

---

[1] Many cultural groups have catastrophic cognitions about sounds heard upon rotation of the joints.

and twisting the shoulders, by rotating the neck, by putting the arms out straight, then rotating them one way then the other. Stretch anywhere in the body you want. [The therapist can do any of the described stretches: rolling the shoulders, rotating the head, and/or extending the arms straight out in front of the body, rotating them in a stretching motion.]

7. *Repeat the contraction and stretching one or two more times if you want.* [The therapist repeats one more time.]

❑ *Arms and hands.* Now let us relax and stretch the arms and hands.

1. *Tighten.* Now tighten both hands, making fists, with a light tension, just barely closing them. Now curl both your arms upward, bringing your forearms to your biceps. You should feel light tension.

2. *Count.* Now hold this position as you count slowly to ten: one, two, three, four, five, six, seven, eight, nine, ten.

3. *Release.* Now let go of the tension.

4. *Positive imagery.* Notice the feeling of warmth in your hands, as if the blood is running smoothly in your arms, all blockages removed.

5. *Stretch the muscle.* Now stretch the arms, for example, by putting the arms straight out, and rotating them, rotating the wrists. [The therapist enacts this stretching.]

6. *Stretch any area of tension.* Wherever you feel tense in your body, do stretching; for example, by rolling and twisting the shoulders, by rotating the neck, by putting the arms out straight, then rotating them one way, then the other. Stretch anywhere in the body you want. [The therapist can do any of the described stretches: rolling the shoulders, rotating the head, and/or

extending the arms straight out in front of the body, rotating them in a stretching motion.]

7. *Repeat the contraction and stretching one or two more times if you want.* [The therapist repeats one more time.]

❑ *The shoulders.* Now let us relax and stretch the shoulders.

1. *Tighten.* Raise your shoulders. It should be a light tension, using just enough force to raise them.

2. *Count.* Now hold this position as you count slowly to ten: one, two, three, four, five, six, seven, eight, nine, ten.

3. *Release.* Now let go of the tension.

4. *Positive imagery.* Notice the feeling of warmth in your body, the release of tension, a slight warmth.

5. *Stretch the muscle.* Now stretch the shoulders by twisting the shoulders. [The therapist enacts this stretching.]

6. *Stretch any area of tension.* Wherever you feel tense in your body, do stretching; for example, by rolling and twisting the shoulders, by rotating the neck, by putting the arms out straight, then rotating them one way, then the other. Stretch however you want. [The therapist can do any of the described stretches: rolling the shoulders, rotating the head, and/or extending the arms straight out in front of the body, rotating them in a stretching motion.]

7. *Repeat the contraction and stretching one more time.*

❑ *The jaw.* Now let us relax and stretch the jaw.

1. *Tighten.* Now tighten your jaw slightly, lightly bringing the teeth together, lightly biting down.

2. *Count.* Now hold this position as you count slowly to ten: one, two, three, four, five, six, seven, eight, nine, ten.

3. *Release.* Now let go of the tension.

4. *Positive imagery.* Notice the feeling of warmth in your face, the release of tension, a slight warmth.

5. *Stretch that muscle.* Now stretch the jaw by opening it wide, moving it from side to side. You can rub this muscle to relax it. [The therapist enacts this stretching and rubs the jaw.]

6. *Stretch any area of tension.* Wherever you feel tense in your body, do stretching; for example, by rolling and twisting the shoulders, by rotating the neck, by putting the arms out straight, then rotating them one way, then the other. Stretch anywhere in the body you want. [The therapist can do any of the described stretches: rolling the shoulders, rotating the head, and/or extending the arms straight out in front of the body, rotating them in a stretching motion.]

7. *Repeat the contraction and stretching one or two more times if you want.* [The therapist repeats one more time.]

◻ *The mouth.* Now let us relax and stretch the mouth.

1. *Tighten.* Now make a pouting motion with the mouth, as if you have just put something very sour in your mouth like a lemon.

2. *Count.* Now hold this position as you count slowly to ten: one, two, three, four, five, six, seven, eight, nine, ten.

3. *Release.* Now let go of the tension.

4. *Positive imagery.* Notice the feeling of warmth in your face, the release of tension, a slight warmth.

5. *Stretch the muscle.* Now open the mouth wide, and move the jaw from side to side, stretching, making facial expressions, moving the lips out. Also, you can take your hand and rub your cheeks to stretch the muscle. Now stretch the mouth by making a broad smile. You can rub the jaw muscle to relax it. [The therapist enacts this stretching.]

6. *Stretch any area of tension.* Wherever you feel tense in your body, do stretching; for example, by rolling and twisting the shoulders, by rotating the neck, by putting the arms out straight, then rotating them one way, then the other. Stretch anywhere in the body you want. [The therapist can do any of the described stretches: rolling the shoulders, rotating the head, and/or extending the arms straight out in front of the body, rotating them in a stretching motion.]

7. *Repeat the contraction, and stretching one or two more times if you want.* [The therapist repeats one more time.]

◻ *The forehead and eyebrows.* Now let us relax and stretch the eyebrow area and forehead.

1. *Tighten.* Now knit your eyebrows, tensing them slightly, feeling the tension.

2. *Count.* Now hold this position as you count slowly to ten: one, two, three, four, five, six, seven, eight, nine, ten.

3. *Release.* Now let go of the tension.

4. *Positive imagery.* Notice the feeling of warmth in your face, the release of tension, a slight warmth.

5. *Stretch that muscle.* Now stretch this area, by raising the eyebrows, letting them down, stretching that area. Take your hand and rub your forehead to relax the muscle. [The therapist enacts this stretching.]

6. *Stretch any area of tension.* Wherever you feel tense in your body, do stretching; for example, by rolling and twisting the shoulders, by rotating the neck, by putting the arms out straight, then rotating them one way, then the other. Anywhere you want. [The therapist can do any of the described stretches: rolling the shoulders, rotating the head, and/or extending the arms straight out in front of the

body, rotating them in a stretching motion.]

7. *Repeat the contraction and stretching one or two more times if you want.* [The therapist repeats one more time.]

□ *The right side of your neck.* Now let us relax and stretch the right side of your neck.

1. *Tighten.* Take your right hand, raise it up, and put it on the side of your head. Push your head against the hand, lightly.

2. *Count.* Now hold this position as you count slowly to ten: one, two, three, four, five, six, seven, eight, nine, ten.

3. *Release.* Now stop pushing the head, and return it to the upright.

4. *Positive imagery.* Notice the feeling of warmth in your body, the release of tension, a slight warmth.

5. *Stretch that muscle.* Now stretch the neck, by rotating the head. If you hear any sounds, do not be concerned. It is just the sound of tendons and muscle; it is just stretching and there is no danger. [The therapist enacts this stretching.]

6. *Stretch any area of tension.* Wherever you feel tense in your body, do stretching; for example, by rolling and twisting the shoulders, by rotating the neck, by putting the arms out straight, then rotating them one way, then the other. Stretch anywhere in the body you want. [The therapist can do any of the described stretches: rolling the shoulders, rotating the head, and/or extending the arms straight out in front of the body, rotating them in a stretching motion.]

7. *Repeat the contraction and stretching one or two more times if you want.* [The therapist repeats one more time.]

□ *The left side of your neck.* Now let us relax and stretch the left side of your neck.

1. *Tighten.* Take your left hand, raise it up, and put it on the side of your head. Push your head against the hand, lightly.

2. *Count.* Now hold this position as you count slowly to ten: one, two, three, four, five, six, seven, eight, nine, ten.

3. *Release.* Now stop pushing the head, and return it to the upright.

4. *Positive imagery.* Notice the feeling of warmth in your body, the release of tension, a slight warmth.

5. *Stretch the muscle.* Now stretch the neck, by rotating the head. If you hear any sounds, do not be concerned. It is just the sound of tendons and muscle; it is just stretching and there is no danger. [The therapist enacts this stretching.]

6. *Stretch any area of tension.* Wherever you feel tense in your body, do stretching; for example, by rolling and twisting the shoulders, by rotating the neck, by putting the arms out straight, then rotating them one way, then the other. Stretch anywhere in the body you want. [The therapist can do any of the described stretches: rolling the shoulders, rotating the head, and/or extending the arms straight out in front of the body, rotating them in a stretching motion.]

7. *Repeat the contraction and stretching one or two more times if you want.* [The therapist repeats one more time.]

□ *Visualization.* Keeping your eyes closed, we now want you to imagine the following.

• *Teaching the Palm Tree Visualization*

Mood determined by attentional object

The images in our minds, what we think about, determine how we feel. Now you will bring your attentional gaze to a good image, a healing image.

Beach-scene visualization

Keeping your eyes closed, imagine the following [the therapist tries to evoke all the senses, as in the following]:

1. You are under a palm tree at the beach on a sunny day.
2. You see near you flowers and fruit-laden trees, with mangoes and other fruit.
3. You see palm fronds [i.e., leaves] swaying in the wind by the sea, the fronds moving in each slight breeze, making a swishing sound, the trunk slightly swaying, the ocean nearby.
4. You see the ocean and its waves, the waves breaking on the shore.
5. You hear the waves crashing on the shore.
6. You hear other ambient nature sounds, the sound of birds singing, of gulls, around you.
7. You hear the most beautiful singing voices of children of all ages, some of them playing the *daf* (a large Persian and Arabic frame drum), layered together.[2] [May also use the example of listening to the most beautiful Quran recitation (e.g., by your favorite Quran reciter[3]); or listening to your favorite *nasheed*, Islamically themed songs often revolving around praising Allah, or the virtues of prophet Muhammad, and/or other religious themes.[4]]

8. You smell the saltiness of the sea, as the waves crash down.
9. You feel the hot sand with your toes, the warm sand under your toes, its heat.
10. You feel the sun's heat and ocean's spray on your skin, you feel the sun on your skin, its heat on your face and body. Then you feel a cool breeze on your skin, the spray coming off the waves.

Palm tree visualization paired with head rotation

1. Envision a palm tree with its large fronds swaying in the wind, near the ocean.
2. Straighten your spine by tightening your stomach muscles slightly at the level of your belly button.
3. Keeping your spine straight, raise your shoulders and count to three very slowly: one, two, three.
4. Drop the shoulders.
5. Straighten the spine again by tightening the muscles in the stomach.
6. Keeping your spine straight, imagine your spine is like the trunk of the palm tree, and your head is like the fronds.
7. Keeping your spine straight, rotate your head on your shoulders.
8. While rotating the head, imagine your head is like the palm fronds circling in the wind, dancing in the breeze, at the end of the trunk, bending this way and that, playing in the wind.[5]
9. While rotating your head, ask that you "be able to adjust to each new situation,

---

[2] Images of layering promote a cognitive set of multi-set flexibility.

[3] The therapist may mention as examples world-famous Quran reciters such as the late Abdul Basit Abdul Samad and Mishary Al Afasy; many practicing Muslims will be aware of these reciters.

[4] *Nasheeds* are immensely popular Islamic-themed songs; they have garnered millions of views on YouTube. Notable *nasheed* singers include Maher Zain and Ahmed Bukhatir, who may be mentioned.

[5] Please note that interoceptive exposure is here introduced into the relaxation protocol. Also, reassociation to the sensation of dizziness is being taught.

just as the palm trunk and palm fronds dance and adjust to each new breeze."

10. Repeat 1 through 9 two more times.

Final stretching

Stretch anywhere you feel tension: your shoulders, your arms, your mouth, your jaw [The therapist demonstrates stretching in any one of these areas. The therapist models how to do the stretching, and the patient imitates. The therapist should discretely observe the patient, to make sure it is done appropriately. If correction is needed, make sure to compliment the patient, and to smile, when making corrections.]

Appendix C   Dysphoria (Anxiety/Depression) Protocol

Whenever you feel anxious, depressed, or tense, you may want to do the following visualization and method of relaxing the body. It will help to relax your mood, to move your mind to a good image, to help you to be more flexible, and to distance yourself from a negative mood.

- **Dysphoria protocol with palm tree visualization**

Palm tree visualization paired with head rotation

1. *Envision a palm tree.* Try to conjure in your mind the image of a palm tree with its large fronds swaying in the wind, near the ocean.
2. *Straight spine.* Tighten your stomach muscles slightly at the level of the belly button, so making your spine straight.
3. *Shoulder raising.* Raise your shoulders.
4. *Counting.* Count to three, slowly.
5. *Drop.* Drop the shoulders.
6. *Straight spine.* Keep your spine straight by tightening the muscles in the stomach.
7. *Pairing of the trunk of the palm tree with the spine, the fronds with the head.* Keeping your spine straight, imagine your spine is like the trunk of the palm tree, and your head is like the fronds.
8. *Head rotation with a straight spine.* Keeping your spine straight, rotate your head on your shoulders.
9. *Visualization of the wind-moved palm fronds.* While rotating the head, think to yourself, the back is like the trunk of the palm, the head like the fronds that dance in the wind.
10. *Pairing with an instructional meaning.* Ask that you "be able to adjust to each new situation, just as the palm fronds are able to dance and adjust to each new breeze."
11. Repeat 1 through 10 two more times.

Final stretching
Stretch anywhere you feel tension:
- ➤ You can roll the shoulders.
- ➤ You can hold out and stretch your arms by rotating them back and forth. [The therapist puts the arms straight forward and rotates them back and forth, then rotates at the wrist.]
- ➤ Stretch wherever you feel tension in your body. [The therapist can stretch other areas too, like the jaw.]

Appendix D   Bad Memory Protocol (Emotion Regulation Toolbox)

Tool for when you have trauma recall. You can do any of the following when you think of the past but don't want to or when distressed for any reason. Some of these methods we have already taught you. These are like a box of "tools" you can use.

Use whichever one you like. Use whichever one you want, whichever one is helpful. They are a set of tools, which you can use in any way you find useful.

We will review multiple times. We will review it many times, so you can remember it.

• Emotion shifts

Try shifting emotions, try different emotions, try different ways of thinking, try changing perspectives. Try some of the following emotions:

Acknowledge having suffered

It did happen. I did suffer. Allow yourself to feel the pain, to let it be, to acknowledge that it did happen and it was hard. Things like that happen in this life.

Compassion

Compassion for all those who have suffered, and compassion for yourself. You should have a feeling of compassion for all those who have suffered and for yourself

Like water flowing from your heart. Having compassion for others and for yourself that flows like "water" from your heart in all directions.

Water and compassion directed to all who have suffered including yourself. Feel this cool water flowing from your heart, first directed towards God, then his prophets, then to the *ummah* (global Muslim community), and then to all beings, a feeling of love and compassion for all beings including yourself.

162

• Comfort the inner child

Tell the inner child, "That was then, this is now; you are now in this place, at this moment, now." Comfort the inner child. Tell the inner child, tell yourself, that you are here [name country and city], on this particular day. You are here, on this day of the week, in this season.[6] Comfort that part of yourself.

[Can mention that the inner child may be soothed by doing *dhikr*; and that the Quran encourages one to call upon God using His different names (see Quran verse 17:110–111), and that he or she may evoke these names of Allah and ponder their deeper meanings to soothe the inner child. Those names of God that make the inner child feel safe should be used, such as *Ar-Rahman* (the Most Merciful), *Al-Wadood* (the Most Loving), *Al-Mumin* (the Granter of Security), *Al-Muhaymin* (the Protecter), *Al-Gafur* (the Forgiving), *Al-Salam* (the Ultimate Provider of Peace), *Al-Muqit* (the Nourisher) and so on (see Table 2 for selected names of God, which may be copied to give to the patient). Another *dhikr* that a patient may say to soothe the inner child is repeating each of three distinct praises of God – *subhanAllah* (glory be to God) thirty-three times, *alhamdulilah* (praise be to God) thirty-three times, *Allahuakbar* (God is the greatest) thirty-four times – all the while using his or her fingers to count (called *tasbeeh*). Also, one can mention to the patient the following verse in the Quran, in which God says, "in the remembrance of God the hearts find rest" (Quran: 13:28),

---

[6] If the patient is in a place where trauma is still occurring, then this will not apply.

a reassurance that the *dhikr* may bring the inner peace and comfort, the cravings of the inner child.]

- **Bring yourself into the present moment with all your senses**

  Come into the moment: Time and place. Try to be aware only of the present moment, here around you, right now, here in [mention country], here in [mention city], to what is around you right now, at this moment.

  Come into the moment: The senses. Try to be aware of what is going around you, with one or more your senses. [The therapist should describe each sense slowly, in some detail, so there is a sense of actually experiencing the sensory modality, a sort of immersion in it. Again, to repeat, it is very important to slow the voice, to deepen the voice, to create a sense of relaxation.]

  ❖ *Visual.* Look out the window at the branches gently swaying, up-and-down or side-to-side. [The therapist points out the window.] Look at the blue color of the sky, the appearance of the clouds, their shape, the way they move, their color.

  ❖ *Sound.* Or listen to the sounds around you. [The therapist points at the ear, and then describes all the ambient sounds: voices, cars passing by, the hum of the air conditioning, the creaking of floorboards or doors; the sound of one's own breathing.]

  ❖ *Tactile.* Or you can feel the coolness or warmth of your skin, and maybe notice the shift in temperature as a slight breeze blows against your skin.

  ❖ *Body motion.*[7] Or you can feel the weight of your arm as you move it upward, the feeling of it moving in space. Without even looking at your

arm or leg, you know its position in space. It is a special skill you have. [The therapist makes such a movement of the arms while describing the motion, moving the arm slowly up and down, bending it. The therapist should close the eyes at one point.]

  ❖ *Olfactory.* Or maybe you smell an odor.

  ❖ *Muscle tension.* Or be aware of any tension, and relax it by stretching it. You might find you have tension in your arm, so you point it out straight, then rotate it from side to side. [The therapist can relax any muscle group: the jaw, opening the mouth wide, massaging the jaw; the shoulders, lifting and moving the shoulders back and forth; the neck, rotating the head.]

- **Dysphoria Protocol**

You can do the following, bringing this image to your mind.

Palm tree visualization paired with head rotation

1. *Envision a palm tree.* Try to conjure in your mind the image of a palm tree with its large fronds swaying in the wind, near the ocean.

2. *Straight spine.* Tighten your stomach muscles slightly, thereby making your spine straight.

3. *Shoulders raised.* Raise your shoulders.

4. *Counting.* Count to three, slowly.

5. *Shoulders dropped.* Drop your shoulders.

6. *Straight spine.* Keep your spine straight by tightening the muscles in your stomach.

7. *Pairing of the palm trunk with the spine and the fronds with the head.* Keeping your spine straight, imagine your spine is like the trunk of the palm tree, and your head is like the fronds at its top.

---

[7] This involves multiple sensory modalities, including kinesthetics.

8. *Head rotation with a straight spine.* Keeping your spine straight, rotate your head on your shoulders.

9. *Visualization of the wind-blown palm fronds.* Imagine your head is like the large palm fronds circling in the wind; that like the palm fronds, your head is dancing in the wind, bending this way and that, playing in the wind.

10. *Pairing with an instructional meaning.* Ask that you "be able to adjust to each new situation, just as the palm fronds are able to adjust to and dance in each new breeze."

11. Repeat 1 through 10 two more times.

• Applied stretching
Relaxing areas of identified tension

You should relax any area of identified tension. Stretch any area you wish to. [At this point, the therapist should sit upright and rotate the head, modeling a relaxation of the neck, and open the mouth wide and stretch and make a side-to-side motion, thereby modeling the relaxation of the mouth and jaw.]

Example of arm-focused stretching by rotation: Shoulder, arm, elbow, wrist, and fingers

Let us use the arm as an example. [The therapist needs to model these actions, while he or she instructs the patient. The aim is to stretch and relax all the joints in the arm, including the shoulder joint, elbow, wrist, and fingers. The therapist should be aware of making motions at those joints, either sequentially or simultaneously, as described below.]

1. Straight-arm rotation stretch
   i. Extend one or both arms in front of the body, straight enough that there is some tension in the elbow.
   ii. Bend back the wrists.

iii. Rotate the straightened arms, once in one direction, until there is a sense of slight tension.
   iv. Hold it there as you count to three, slowly.
   v. Rotate the arms in the other direction until there is some sense of tension.
   vi. Hold it there as you count to three, slowly.
   vii. Repeat this a couple times. You can do it with one or both arms.

2. Wrist rotation stretch
   i. Bend the arm a little (approximately 45 degrees).
   ii. Rotate the wrists, one way and then the other, with one or both wrists.

3. Finger wiggle stretch
   i. Straighten the fingers, feeling some tension in the joints, arch them back to create more tension.
   ii. With the fingers straight, wriggle them back and forth.
   iii. Do this with one or both hands.

4. Repeat any part you like, such as the wrist rotation
   i. Bend the arm at the elbow slightly.
   ii. Rotate the wrists, one way and then the other.

• Abbreviated version of the Trauma Protocol

Whenever you are anxious, or have trauma recall, you can choose the part you like of those things we have shown you. For example, try any of the following:

Try different emotions

For example, feel compassion and love for yourself and others.

Bring yourself into the moment

Attend to what is happening around you right now, using all your senses:

what you see outside the window, how the wind feels on your skin, what you smell.

Try to stretch the body

Stretch wherever you feel tense. Open your mouth and move it from side to side, straighten and rotate the arm. [The therapist should enact these motions.]

Do something you like

You may want to do something you like. For example, you may want to take a walk or watch television.

Appendix E   Anger Protocol (Anger Toolbox)

The following are some tools you can use when you are angry.

- **Religious ideas about anger**
  - True strength. Several narrations by the prophet Muhammad in which he stresses that true virtue lies in not getting angry, and that true strength is not physical strength (i.e., being muscular) but controlling anger.
  - Sit or lie down. The prophet Muhammad advised his followers in a famous narration, "When one of you becomes angry while standing, he should sit down. If the anger leaves him, well and good; otherwise he should lie down."[8]
  - *Wudhu.* When angry you can do *wudhu* (ritualistic washing of limbs).
  - Change location, leaving the place in which you were angered.

- **Dysphoria protocol when you are angry**

If you become angry, you can stretch the shoulders and neck and bring to mind a good thing.

➢ Palm tree visualization paired with head rotation

1. *Envision a palm tree.* Try to conjure in your mind the image of a palm tree with its large fronds swaying in the wind, near the ocean.
2. *Straight spine.* Tighten your stomach muscles slightly at the level of the belly button, so making your spine straight.
3. *Shoulders raised.* Raise your shoulders.
4. *Counting.* Count to three, slowly.

5. *Shoulders dropped.* Drop the shoulders.
6. *Straight spine.* Keep your spine straight by tightening the muscles in the stomach.
7. *Pairing of the trunk of the palm tree with the spine, the fronds with the head.* Keeping your spine straight, imagine your spine is like the trunk of the palm tree, and your head is like the fronds.
8. *Head rotation with a straight spine.* Keeping your spine straight, rotate your head on your shoulders.
9. *Visualization of the wind-blown palm fronds.* While rotating the head, think to yourself, the back is like the trunk of the palm, the head like the fronds that dance in the wind.
10. *Pairing with an instructional meaning.* Ask that you "be able to adjust to each new situation, just as the palm fronds are able to dance and adjust to each new breeze."
11. Repeat 1 through 10 two more times

➢ *Final stretching.* Stretch anywhere you feel tension: your shoulders your arms, your mouth, your jaw.

- **Stretch any area of tension**
You could try the following [The therapists models the following]:
  - Stretch the muscles in the face
    ➢ Relax the jaw
      ▪ Stretch the jaw, by opening the mouth wide and moving the jaw from side to side.

---

[8] In Sunan Abi Dawud.

- Use your hand to massage the jaw to stretch and relax its muscles.

➢ Relax the forehead
  - Stretch the eyebrow area, the forehead, by wrinkling and releasing the forehead.
  - Use the hand to massage the forehead to stretch its muscles.

○ Relax the neck and shoulders
  ➢ Massage the muscles in any area where you feel tension, as in the neck.
  ➢ Roll the shoulders.

○ Stretch the arm
  ➢ Stretch the arms
    - Put one or both arms straight out, until there is tightness, and bend back the wrists.
    - Rotate the arms, all the way in one direction, then all the way in the other, feeling the sense of stretching.

  ➢ Stretch the wrists
    - Bend the arm slightly, and then rotate the wrist, feeling the stretching.

  ➢ Stretch the fingers
    - Straighten the fingers and wiggle them.

Embodying metaphors

While doing these exercises, you should think the following while doing the stretching:

➢ "As I become more flexible in my body, may I become flexible in my thoughts, in my emotions, may I know how to adjust to each new situation." [Or, "Oh Allah may I become more flexible in my body, may I become more flexible in my thoughts, in my emotions, may I know how to adjust to each new situation."]

- **Using an instructional proverb: Gaining a hundred days of happiness**
Don't forget the old proverb: "If you control your anger one time, you gain a hundred days of happiness."

- **Distance yourself from mood**
Distance yourself from anger. Try to be far from your mood, pull your heart back from your mood, just watch your mood. Distance yourself from your anger.
Observe anger's effects on the body and mind. Just observe anger's effects on your mind and body, on your emotions.
Cloud-as-anger comparison. Watch your anger as if it is a cloud in the sky. Soon it will pass out of your mind, like a cloud passes from the sky.

- **Delay action**
Delay action to avoid regret. If you act when you are angry, you may well regret later what you have said or done.
Wait to act. Wait until the anger has lessened before making a decision about what to do.

- **Make no decisions when angry**
Not seeing clearly when angry. When we are angry, we don't see things clearly. When you are angry, you can't analyze clearly, and you will make mistakes.
Making decision when calm again. Wait until you are calm before you do anything or decide anything. If you do something when angry, you will regret it later. Wait until you are cool in the heart before making a decision.

- **Don't be a slave to your emotions**

Don't be a slave to your emotions. Distance yourself from the emotion, consider other ways of reacting.

- **Consider other emotions**
  - ○ *Compassion.* Maybe you should feel compassion for the other person, feel sorry for them, hope they gain wisdom.

- **Consider other causes for the other persons' actions (reframing)**

Remember, they may act as they do because of their own misery, their own problems, their own suffering, their own ignorance. Try to feel compassion for all beings.

- **Be a good example for your children (Use this example if the patient has children)**

Others will do as you do. Remember, your children will do what you do, not what you say. If you act angry, if you drink, your children will do the same: they will express anger quickly with others and will get into trouble.

If you improve, others will follow your example. Even if you used to get very angry in the past, if you now learn to control your anger, your children will learn that one can change and improve. It's an important lesson you can teach your children.

- **Living in the moment with all the senses**

When you are angry, you can try any form of multisensorial living-in-the-moment practice with all the senses.

Choose the one you like. You can choose any sensory channel. [The therapist then models the following, by describing these things, as in colors or leaf movement

seen out the window. It is best to speak slowly in order to increase relaxation.]:

- ➤ *Visual.* Pay attention to images around you:[9]
  - ○ Leaves
    - ■ *Leaf movements.* You may pay attention to how the leaves move in the wind, or how branches move.
    - ■ *Leaf shapes.* Note the different shapes of leaves – pointy, round, jagged, flat, curved – or the shapes of branches.
    - ■ *Leaf color.* Note the different color of leaves, bright green, light green, yellow, or the different colors of branches.

  - ○ Clouds
    - ■ *Cloud movements.* You may pay attention to how the clouds move across the sky.
    - ■ *Cloud shapes.* Note the different shapes of the clouds – puffy, streaky, round.
    - ■ *Cloud colors.* Note the colors of the clouds, with their whites and greys, or the colors of the sky.

- ➤ *Sounds.* Or you can pay attention to the sounds around you.
- ➤ *Body motion (kinesthetic).* Or you can pay attention to the way your arms or legs or other body parts feel as they move through space, the heaviness of your arms or legs as they move. [The therapist should move an arm, describing its multidirectional movement in space.]

---

[9] If there are not many leaves or branches, the sky and clouds can be used: how clouds move in the sky, the shape of clouds, the color of clouds and sky.

➢ *Tactile.* Or you can pay attention to the feel of the wind on your skin, any skin sensations.

➢ *Breath.* Or you can pay attention to your breath, the way your breath goes in, then out, through your nose.

➢ *Smells.* Be aware of smells. Maybe you want to hold a flower and smell it, or smell a favorite cologne or perfume.

➢ *Muscular.* Or you can pay attention to any tension in your body, and once you identify it, relax it. [The therapist models stretching a body zone, like the shoulders.]

• Performing loving kindness

You can practice having loving kindness. It is a way to practice having an emotion other than anger.

Water and cooling imagery

❑ Upon leaving today, as you walk along, practice projecting sublime love to God, love to his prophets, and then love to all beings.

❑ Loving kindness is a way to practice having a positive emotion.

❑ Direct love to Allah (or God) (a type of ultimate love); and thereafter his prophets (e.g., prophet Muhammad, and prophets such as Adam, Noh [i.e., Noah], Ibrahim [i.e., Abraham], Musa [i.e., Moses], and Eisa [i.e., Jesus]).

❑ Direct love and kindness to your parents (e.g., starting with your mother and then father) and then the rest of your family.[10]

❑ Direct love and kindness to the *ummah* (global Muslim community) and then all beings.[11]

❑ Direct love and kindness to yourself.

❑ Imagine love flowing from your heart, like a cooling water.

❑ Imagine the water going out from your heart in all directions.

❑ Imagine that the water extinguishes all anger.

❑ Wish that all beings be happy.

❑ Wish that all beings be free from anger.

❑ Wish that all beings have wisdom.

❑ Imagine loving kindness flowing from your heart to all beings, like a water flowing from your heart.

❑ Practice projecting a feeling of sublime love to God and love and kindness to all beings as you go home, and during the next week. [Could mention here that one may supplicate for others (e.g., asking God to forgive them); e.g., mention that the Quran stresses the importance of supplicating for one's parents in particular: "My Lord, have mercy upon them [my parents] as they brought me up [when I was] small," (17:24), and that the Prophet encouraged the act of supplicating for others in general (a sign of mercy); e.g., he said "no Muslim supplicates for his brother behind his back but that the angel says: And for you the same,"[12] and "none of you has faith until he loves for his brother or neighbour what he loves for himself," and "Allah will not be merciful to those who are not merciful to mankind." One could mention the importance of forgiving others if they have done you wrong; like prophet

---

[10] The Quran stresses the importance of showing parents mercy, especially the mother; for instance, "lower to them [i.e., your parents] the wing of humility out of mercy and say, 'My Lord, have mercy upon them as they brought me up [when I was] small,'" and "We [i.e., God] have enjoined upon man [to take good care] for his parents. His mother carried him, [increasing her] in weakness upon weakness, and his weaning is in two years. Be grateful to Me [i.e., God] and to your

parents." These Quranic verses and sayings of the Prophet may be mentioned to patients.

[11] This order of showing love and kindness is consistent with the Prophet's teachings that Muslims globally belong to a special brotherhood/sisterhood (*ummah*).

[12] Found in the Muslim collection.

Muhammad (the role model for Muslims), who after he was physically abused said, "my Lord, forgive my people for they do not know"[13]; and as the Quran states that Muslims are those "who restrain [their] anger and who pardon the people and Allah loves the doers of good" (3:134). Finally, could mention here that the patient may make *tauba* for himself or herself (i.e., asking God for forgiveness).]

Enjoyable activity: Multisensorial drinking of tea or coffee

You should do something you like. You may want to drink tea or coffee with all your senses, as we have taught you, and at the same time, look out the window, being aware of all the things going on out there, using all your senses.

Wall push-ups

If you feel angry, you can do the wall push-ups, or some other form of exercise, like taking a walk.

Do stretching

If you feel angry, you may want to stretch. You can stretch in any of the ways we taught you. For example, you may roll the shoulders or stretch the jaw, or do any of the stretches in the handout.

---

[13] Found in the Muslim collection.

Index